December 2004

For my Fellow Travelers,
Steve + Nancy —

Elizabeth Loewald

Elizabeth Loewald

SIGHTING ANTON PAVLOVICH

Hermitage Publishers

2004

Loewald Elizabeth
SIGHTING ANTON PAVLOVICH
Essay

Library of Congress Cataloging-in-Publication Data:

Loewald, Elizabeth.
Sighting Anton Pavlovich / Elizabeth Loewald
p. cm.
Includes bibliographical references and index
ISBN 1-55779-149-X (cl: alk. Paper) – ISBN 1-55779-148-1 (pbk.: alk. paper.)
1. Chekhov, Anton Pavlovich, 1860-1904—Career in medicine.
2. Chekhov, Anton Pavlovich, 1860-1904—Health. 3. Tuberculosis—Patients—Russia—Biography. 4. Authors, Russian—19th century—Biography. I. Title.

PG3458.Z9M435 2004
891.72'3—dc22
[B] 2004054117

Cover design by Mikhail Belomlinsky

Published by Hermitage Publishers
P.O. Box 310
Tenafly, N.J. 07670, USA
Tel. (201) 894-8247; Fax (201) 894-5591
E-mail: yefimovim@aol.com

The entire Hermitage Publishers catalog is available on the Internet:
http://www.Hermitagepublishers.com

CONTENTS

For Hans

Preface

One hundred years have passed since Anton Pavlovich Chekhov was buried in the Novodevichie Cemetery of Moscow. His short stories and plays are perennials—not short lived annuals, as some contemporary critics dismissed them—and so his gifts are not lost to us. His works come in and out of fashion. They, as well as his life, are reinterpreted by the light of current social, political and psychological insights. Interest in him and neglect have cycled also in different ways in different countries. His own countrymen, fellow subjects of the Tsar, hailed him or denigrated him, in his lifetime. The USSR co-opted him—collected and treasured his archive, replaced many of his paragraphs black penciled earlier by the Tsar's censors—but then newly deleted others. Meanwhile in England, he became role model to many writers and intellectuals. The brevity, atmosphere, the human truth of his works, were beloved. In the 1920s, Constance Garnett translated many of his stories with great fidelity to his voice. Virginia Woolf analyzed his works and methods with admiration. In 1988, at the age of eighty-eight, V.S.Pritchett published a literary and biographical study, *Chekhov, a Spirit Set Free*. Professor Donald Rayfield of the University of London gave scholars and readers everywhere the gift of a fulsome, carefully researched 1997 biography, *Anton Chekhov, a Life*. This list only begins the naming of fine interpreters of Chekhov, and omits many whose criticism has been fresh and valuable in many parts of the world. Charles Du Bos, a French critic in the 1920s, has stood out for me. He published observations that are unique, about Chekhov. He never attempted an entire book, he said, because he felt he still had not understood enough. He said, "Chekhov stops when what might remain to be said could not be at the same time new and true . . . [he] is never inclined to detain [the reader] with anything that the reader can make out or imagine for himself." He wrote: "Chekhov's originality is that he shows the depths at the very instant when the surface reflects them..."[1]

As reader and playgoer, I met Chekhov here in America. Constance Garnett's translations of his stories reached us on the west coast of the United States, where I was an adolescent. "The Cherry Orchard" was produced in Berkeley at the University of California: moving, and very foreign. I came East for medical school and ensuing years. As Chekhov has been forgotten and rediscovered in various time periods, various countries—so for me personally he would vanish for years at a time. Then a production of one of his plays, or an article about him in a journal, or a new collection of his stories, came to remind me of his great value. His world deserved, more and more, to be visited. He was especially corrective to over-complicating life. His friend Maksim Gorki said of him, "Beautifully simple himself, he loved everything simple, genuine, sincere, and he had a peculiar way of making other people simple."[2] His works also have this effect on readers.

Along with readerly appreciation, I developed in later years a special feeling for Chekhov the individual. I believe this is because he followed, in life, some paths that I have also followed. Over a hundred years ago, he made a career not only in literature but in medicine. He was ill with tuberculosis, as I have been. I was curious—how did he feel about these things? Why did they happen to him? I myself have had a career in medicine, as a psychiatrist. I have been a writer in some periods of my life—enough to be acquainted with experiences and pitfalls of that choice. I had tuberculosis for six years in my twenties. No medicine to cure consumption had yet been discovered—for Chekhov, nor for me. I was in a sanatorium, and he was not. Otherwise, I experienced the non-specific palliative care that he too, skeptically, received; and the ominously unpredictable course of the disease.

These are reasons I have wanted to know him; and to present my thoughts and gathered information. Literary criticism I have left to many, better-qualified others. So only a few of his works are mentioned here, when they are clearly pertinent. I am an 'ordinary reader' of Chekhov; emboldened a little by his remark in a letter to Suvorin, "You and I like ordinary people..."[3] His relationships with family members, friends, lovers, a wife, I have also not tried to illuminate in particulars. Professor Rayfield, in *Anton Chekhov, a Life*, has presented the most solidly researched information to date about all this.

One of my focal points is the intersection of Dr. Chekhov's career as a doctor with his literary career. Another is his tubercular illness, intersecting with the lines of all else in his life. The time periods, circumstances, interweavings, surely can help us to understand the man, and his stories and plays. I've tried, too, to include some perspectives which have developed in medical thought, and in thinking about tuberculosis, since Chekhov's time. They may enlighten us about him retrospectively. Chekhov was a man much interested in the development of knowledge. He wrote with a long view, and a close view. He had both scientific and poetic standards for his own thought. So I have organized this book in the same spirit; 'sighting' him in ways that became meaningful to me as my own life progressed.

This journey to Chekhov and the review of my own life course seem to intertwine. In Chapter I, I begin with Chekhov's story as a "Russian Tale": his life in a foreign place, in a more portentous and magical time than I knew in my own youthful home. In later adolescence, I began to suspect that myths, so filled with truth, need the supplement of real experiences and disciplines to bring the truth to life.

Those perspectives are used in the next chapters, for exploring Chekhov's history, his photographs, his physical and psychical realities. Then finally, I place a short fiction about Chekhov's first hospitalization. Stories, in the end, suggest the most meaning.

Much help was given me along the way. I especially thank Stephen Farrand, my Russian teacher. Also, my friend Tatyana Schneller, who sat with me, patient or enthusiastic, through my halting reading aloud of many works of Chekhov. She brought along the richness of her native-born Russian—and intimate knowledge of many things Russian, small and big.

I thank Stephen and his wife Nancy for traveling to Russia with me. We saw for ourselves St. Petersburg and Moscow and Yalta. In Moscow, I am especially grateful to Alevtina Kuzicheva, who gave us her time and her kind expert guidance to places Chekhov frequented .

Bella Z. Berson, now retired from the post of Director of the Medical Library at Yale University, was an indispensable friend. She sifted electronic files for the books in Russian or English, which I wanted to read— then helped me through formidable systems of the Yale University Library to find them.

Through it all, in Portland, Maine, my writer friend Alfred DePew encouraged me to stand by the unorthodox format of this book. I appreciate that.

I.
A Russian Tale

One January, a healthy baby boy was born in the provincial city of Taganrog, on the Sea of Azov. He was named Anton Pavlovich, at his christening in the town's Russian Cathedral. This was a century and a half ago. Many things were different from what you and I know. The language, the food, the names of birds and flowers and trees; the severity of life under a Tsar—and, for example, it was not surprising then that Anton's father believed it was a portent, when just before the baby's birth the dome of the Church of St. Michael was struck by lightning and caught fire.

In Anton's family were a father, mother, and two older brothers. They lived in a one-story house with a red wooden roof, ornamented with burdock, nettles, buttercups, and a mass of pleasant flowers.[1] In the cottage were five small rooms. A Russian nurse was hired to help the ailing mother: Anton's father could afford this at the time because the grocery store he owned was doing well. The nurse, like himself, was an ex-serf. Russian serfs had just been liberated by the Tsar's reform decree. And even earlier, a few persistent ones, like Anton's grandfather, had been able to buy their freedom from the landowners.

The baby grew well. Four more children were born to the parents after Anton. The family moved to a larger house on a more prestigious street, when the boy was five, to befit his father's status as 'meshchanin', or petit bourgeois. Father's dignity as citizen was very important to him. A serf in childhood, he wanted full rank and trappings as citizen. He was a zealously religious man. He had become choirmaster at the Cathedral, and alderman of the Police Authority as well.

He moved the family again when Anton was nine, to a two-story brick house with living quarters and room for an expanded business. The shop was at the edge of town, on the corner of a busy avenue. It had a drawing room upstairs with a piano; where prosperous customers could drink tea with the proprietor and relax. In truth, the building was only rented. And the living quarters, in back of the fine shop, were tiny and dank. The family, several tenants, and the shop boys, were crowded there into a few small rooms. The kitchen had no running water. It stank, and was infested with cockroaches.

Family misfortunes began to multiply. The grocery store did poorly as business patterns changed in this trade-route town. Father had heavy debts now. Then Anton's baby sister died, at the age of two, when Anton was eleven. His mother mourned deeply. Already a timid woman, dominated and policed by her husband, she sank into a sadness that seldom lifted. Then father suffered a sharp blow. He was dismissed as choirmaster of the Russian Cathedral in Taganrog. He found a lesser musical post at the town's Greek monastery, which had begun to offer liturgical services in Russian as well as Greek. But the existing choir had no altos or sopranos. He commandeered his three oldest sons to fill this void. They began several years of long practices and performances under the hand of their father—that same hand which more and more frequently beat them for their transgressions at home. There were early matins, masses, interminable Easter services—summer and winter, morning, or night. With all this singing, with helping long hours now in the store, with eagle-eyed paternal oversight of their school grades and their behavior (and little help from an exhausted mother), Anton and his brothers lived grimly, at home.

It was different outside these walls, however. For some hours of the day, and especially in school vacations, the brothers were free to roam the countryside around their town. Anton fished and swam. He was expert at catching finches:

sold some of them for small change, in town. They combed for shells of the long-receded sea, in the old cemetery. When Anton was eleven, he and his oldest brother hitched a ride in summer on an oxcart and crossed the steppe, to visit their grandfather. The visit was brief, the grandfather inhospitable—but the two boys made a cheerful way home , walking and hitching, relishing new places.

Anton Pavlovich showed an early natural interest in theater. He was comedian and jokester among his school friends. At home, as a boy, he directed and starred in plays that brought friends and neighbors to the family living room, and made even his dour parents smile. In his tableaus, notables of the town were hilariously recognizable. His siblings were his co-actors—in this, as in most of their sufferings and pleasures, they collaborated. Anton was the leader, in theater. As he reached age ten or eleven, he quietly became dominant too in the domestic rank of the brothers. His oldest brother had teased and tormented him in earlier years, but by now Anton was not intimidated. He also stood up to their father with dignity. He was sometimes given foreman authority over the others in daily family matters.

Anton Pavlovich found more and more compelling pastimes during his adolescence. Their town, which had a proud past, had still a lively present. The town gymnasia he attended was, for the provinces, an unusually good one. (It had been chosen by the Tsar's Minister of Education to be an 'example of a conservative, classical education'.) He learned there: both from books, and from much lively political discussion that escaped the ear of the Minister. School was his haven. Corporal punishment was forbidden there. Students were treated with respect and even understanding. Anton was not an avid scholar, he simply passed his examinations, to be sure to reach the University. The school friends he found were most important to his wider education. He, and with him his brothers, was invited to the homes of schoolmates whose fathers were affluent Czech and Russian merchants. He had grown tall and handsome. His still-round face had a distinct peasant cast; his clothes were not elegant, but always neat. His manners were exquisite. His humor, tact, intelligence, won him his welcome. He took pleasure in the company of the well bred young daughters of the merchants, and they found him most attractive.

At the same time, Anton was exploring elsewhere in town. He lost his virginity in the town brothel at thirteen. He and his brothers also learned how to sneak into the provincial theater, well swathed in large overcoats , or under cover of darkness. Sometimes their theater-loving uncle took them. (This was strictly forbidden, both by their fierce religious father and by the political authorities at the gymnasia.) He saw *La Belle Helene*, *Hamlet*, and much else. Now he mounted a family performance of Gogol's *Government Inspector* at home, playing the mayor himself.

So Anton, by late adolescence, had talents and some accomplishments. His family, however, was in trouble.

They had fallen into real poverty. The family moved to a smaller house, and cut back further on food and clothing. Father made attempts to shore up his business with extra stalls, longer hours—but creditors were at his heels. Anton's older brothers had managed to get to the University in Moscow, though they were nearly penniless there. Now father joined them. A year later, he called all the family but Anton to come to him in Moscow. Anton was left at sixteen to finish his last two years of gymnasia. Surviving as he best could, he was also charged with fending off father's creditors, and salvaging some of the belongings they'd had to leave behind. Letters from Moscow described his family's miserable state. A typical message from father to Anton read, "Mama was expecting 20 rubles from you. When she heard that only 12 had been sent, she burst into floods of bitter tears."[2]

Anton sent them a few rubles fairly regularly. He lived with a family friend, in return for tutoring the host's children. His social life and his scholarship began to flourish. He missed his family painfully; but he made the most of these two years. By age eighteen, he had decided to have a medical career. He won a city council scholarship of twenty-five rubles a month. Then he was off, too, to Moscow.

There are two important points to note, before we continue Anton's story.

First, it was while living apart from his family, between the ages of sixteen and nineteen, that Anton articulated his life goals. He defined his ethical priorities clearly, then, for his years to come. These were not church-given rules: Anton and his siblings abandoned organized religion early. They were intensely personal, distilled from his own experience to date. He said he valued above all his personal freedom and dignity. He determined to be respectful, gentle, compassionate in his dealings—but never servile. He would protect his aesthetic sensibility; respect his own talents. He would avoid violence in all its forms.

The second point may have gone unnoticed by Anton himself. One day during his childhood, the angel of death caught sight of him, while happening to fly over the region on various errands. The angel glided down closer to inspect the boy. Then and there he listed Anton for an early death.

Anton looked to be a healthy boy. The potential for premature death was everywhere at hand, however. Tuberculosis abounded in Russia. And in Anton's family, the tubercle bacillus thrived. His lovable, talented uncle died of the disease when Anton was seven. His infant sister died when she was only two. His mother had active tuberculosis at the time of Anton's birth; and her sister had already succumbed to it.

Anton continued to grow sturdily. When he was fifteen, happily visiting a friend's Cossack ranch in summertime, there came a first sign of trouble. After swimming in a cold river there, he developed a sudden fever, and collapsed. His life was probably saved by a nearby Jewish innkeeper who brought Anton through that night with mustard plasters, cold compresses, and tender care. Next day, they carried Anton to the doctor in town who diagnosed 'peritonitis'—cause unknown.

This illness seemed to awaken Anton. He decided that fall to study to become a doctor. To that end, he began to do better in school—particularly in the study of German, the 'medical language'. And only a year or two later, as described, he saw fit to define principles to live by. This is sometimes done by soldiers, even the very young, before they go to battle.

Anton Pavlovich took on the responsibilities of a grown man when he arrived at his family's basement apartment in Moscow. With a little help from his brothers and sister, he scrabbled for money to support them all. Most of his scholarship went for this—as did the rent paid by fellow medical students he brought as boarders—and after awhile, money he earned writing short comic stories for magazines and journals. He improved family morale by insisting on decent behavior from his demanding older brothers, when they visited their parents. Meanwhile he instructed his younger siblings in the ethical habits he himself tried to follow. He was gentle with his mother, and respectful but in charge, with his father. However, he could combine all this with a free-roving life as a medical student—just as he had mixed his earlier working childhood with outside interests and explorations. Medical students can by tradition be heavy drinkers, sexual adventurers, carousers by night—so long as they appear in the assigned clinics by day. Anton Pavlovich lived all this. Even more attractive to him were the new artist and writer companions of his older brothers, who became his lifelong friends.

In medical school, Anton Pavlovich came to understand and love the scientific approach to truth. He also relished clinical work—his observant, principled nature was well honed for this already. After graduating, he hung out his shingle in Moscow and hoped to develop a full practice, to make a good living (as his mother had long hoped). In a very few years, however, it was plain that he drew mostly impecunious patients, in Moscow, and even poorer ones from the peasantry around his summer country house. He wanted to practice independently and as he chose: neither needing the favor of the gentry, nor exhausting himself for very little money in a provincial 'zemstvo' hospital. So he continued to dash off short stories for the magazines, in the down moments of his consulting room. His literary work—sent in under a pseudonym—was soon noticed. By the age of twenty-five, he was published in a prestigious St. Petersburg daily. At twenty-six, his work was praised by a famous older Russian writer; then by a powerful St. Petersburg publisher. These men helped and inspired him. He continued to practice medicine. But also, he began to write more slowly, seriously, innovatively—and under his own name. At age twenty-eight, Anton Pavlovich won the Pushkin Prize for literature. He now was seeing some of his early plays produced, in Moscow and St. Petersburg.

The angel of death meanwhile went about his business. He took tens of thousands of Russian lives in these years by means of cholera, starvation, drink . . . and he spared as many others. He felled Tsar Alexander II by assassination. We know in hindsight, that the angel had allotted Anton just sixteen years more, after he received the Pushkin Prize. But before that, when Anton Pavlovic was twenty-five, he suffered a first severe hemorrhage from the right lung. He was sitting in a courtroom at the time, following a famous fraud trial to report in a prestigious newspaper. In the next years there were many lesser hemorrhages, most often in the spring. He coughed sometimes incessantly. His speaking voice grew ever weaker.

Outwardly, Anton Pavlovich paid little mind. He conducted his public and family life as though impervious to illness. He provided city dwellings and country estates for the family's shelter. He practiced medicine; traveled; wrote, and grew famous. In letters to a few trusted friends, Anton Pavlovich did express worry about his own health. He spoke of a foreshortened life. He described his symptoms—but firmly denied the likeliest diagnosis. Nor did he allow any doctor to examine him.

Some marks of his early poverty, abuse, and yearning for affection, persisted into manhood. Thus, he loved women, but seemed afraid of the dangers of intimacy and would not marry. Tangles, disappointments, approaches and retreats, loneliness, boredom and restlessness, often depleted him. In guarding his independence he sometimes hurt friends, or neglected them. He would not stoop to apology—but Anton Pavlovich clearly judged his own behavior, and then struggled even harder to prove himself in some other direction. Notably, at age twenty-nine, he suddenly decided to journey six thousand miles by land and sea to Siberia, to bear witness as a physician to the regime's inhuman treatment of its prisoners there. He was exhilarated by the prospect. His health was poor before he started, and deteriorated soon after he returned. His family and friends protested when he undertook this grueling trip; but Anton Pavlovich did not listen.

Death had taken one of Anton's older brothers by tuberculosis when Anton was twenty-nine. The last illness, slow and harrowing, occurred in Anton's house, where he had long been serving as his brother's harassed doctor and nurse. At the end he could not endure it. He'd left home overnight just at the time of his brother's death. His family noticed that among the mourners, only Anton did not cry. He was irritable and depressed for months. He only revived, in fact, by planning his trip to Siberia.

On return from there, until he was thirty-seven years old and in spite of constant illness, Anton Pavlovich flourished in many ways. With money enough from his writing, he found a country estate that pleased his family and allowed for some of his oldest pleasures—fishing, gardening, observing nature in all its aspects. He could hold open house for his friends, but also sequester himself to write and think. Anton Pavlovich wrote many stories there. He traveled to Moscow, when well enough, for productions of his plays. There, charming, lively actresses showered him with affection and adulation. These light hearted and non-binding affairs were most agreeable to him.

Then in March of his thirty-eighth year, Anton Pavlovich was struck seriously by illness. He hemorrhaged from the lung so suddenly, profusely, publicly, while dining in a Moscow restaurant, that he could not avoid hospitalization. Respected specialists examined him at long last. A diagnosis of pulmonary tuberculosis was firmly established. Anton Pavlovich was ordered to avoid the harsh winters of Moscow—and even of the countryside of his estate near the city—from then on. He must move south.

He lived seven more years. Most of these he spent in a house he built for himself, his sister and his mother, on a hill by the Black Sea. His body weakened gradually; he became frail and thin, much aged, for a man in his prime. In letters, and in his writer's notebook, he described the loneliness he felt in this beautiful southern 'prison'. He complained that life had lost its savor. Still, he used the strength he had for writing, for tending his southern garden, for friendship, for favorite humanitarian projects—as usual.

Or not as usual. It was as though Anton Pavlovich in this inescapable illness dug deeper into life. From this, he found nourishment to flower before his harsh winter to come. In spite of physical weakness, he produced some of his finest literary work in Yalta.

Those last plays and stories which Anton Pavlovich wrote in his study by the Black Sea were hard labor for him. To readers and viewers, however, they seemed and still seem effortlessly crafted; vivid, true reflections of life precisely as he observed it.

And Anton Pavlovich married. For the first time, three years before his death, he found it possible to give his heart to a woman. They hoped to have a child. That did not happen—but Anton could experience at the end a conscious wish for fatherhood which he had always denied.

The dark angel was poised to stop Anton's heart and declare his last breath, on a July night when Anton was forty-four. In previous days, Anton Pavlovich had had hours of severe pain, labored breathing, lack of sleep—but also brief periods of hope and pleasure. The morning before his death, he invented a comic story for his wife and they laughed together. Even moments before his death—after saying clearly, "I am dying"—he accepted the glass of champagne his doctor offered, and quietly drank it. He said, "I haven't had champagne for a long time". Then he rolled onto his side, in the bed, and died instantly.[3]

A glass of champagne was always offered, in those days, by the physician to the dying patient, if the latter was a medical colleague. Anton Pavlovich may have presented such a glass to doctor/patients himself. In this way the physician could say without words a farewell to a fellow healer—salute their having tried, together, though they'd been defeated. It was a toast to the savor of life and to the sorrow of leaving it. The angel did allow time for this to happen.

II.
Photographs

Names, dates, faces. Given these, we can believe that all this really happened. Chekhov's biographers have provided us well with photographs, and I choose among them some to describe for you in this chapter.

Anton Pavlovich Chekhov was born in Taganrog, Russia, by the Sea of Azov, in January 1860. His grandfather—serf, then freed man, in the Voronezh province of Ukraine—was Egor Mikhailovich Chekhov. Anton's father was Pavel Egorovich Chekhov, and his mother, Evgenia Iakovlevna, was a daughter of the merchant Iakov Morozov. Anton and his brothers and sisters, by Russian custom, all received the patronymic middle name Pavlovich or Pavlovna. For the western reader, that can serve as a reminder of Pavel's imprint on his children's lives. In order of birth, Anton's older brothers were Aleksandr and Kolya, the younger siblings Vanya, Masha, Misha; and Evgenia, who died in early childhood. Baby Evgenia's name especially evokes her mother Evgenia's deep sorrow at her namesake's death.

Since we can never see or talk to these people, or to any others in Anton Pavlovich's life, we turn to photographs. Chekhov himself treasured photographs. He hung the pictures of his friends and heroes to contemplate, on the walls of his studies. Here are a few of the persons in his life as I observe them—and that, too, filtered through the choices of the various biographers whose books include them. Despite filters, nevertheless, we can read the faces.

Here is a formal Chekhov family portrait from 1874, just before Aleksandr graduated from the Taganrog gymnasia. Anton, Kolya, and tall Aleksandr are all wearing their dark school uniforms with military buttons. This garb is interesting because of two anecdotes about it. One concerns the difficulty the Chekhov family had to raise money for the boys' required uniforms. Without the uniform, they were not allowed at school. The other tells of the fine basis Anton's uniform gave him, as a boy, for dressing as Gogol's mayor, or as a military figure, in home theatricals. He needed only to add a sword, a sash and a hat. Misha and little cousin Georgi have on their best suits. Anton's mother and Aunt Ludmilla wear long, shiny black dresses with fine black edgings and white collars. Young Masha looks less funereal but in her Sunday best, in a white pinafore. Pavel and his brother Mitrofan have neat black suits and well trimmed beards. Mitrofan's beard is black. Pavel's is large and quite white, though his moustache is dark still.

Every face here is solemn. That may be an artifact, of course, of photographic methods of the day. A long exposure time discouraged smiling; and the professional photographer arranged his subjects strictly. Here you see many slender hands arranged in an artful way. Aleksandr's is across his chest, at an odd latitude. Mitrofan's is laid chastely on his wife's shoulder. Masha is allowed to lace her hands around her father's forearm; while Pavel and Evgenia, though their chairs are turned slightly towards each other, bend their wrists so that their hands fall away from each other, like decorous nesting birds. Pavel looks imposing and rather melancholy. In all his photographs he appears so. This is a man who in his twenties designed and wore a signet ring inscribed, "Everywhere is a desert to the lonely man." Evgenia's gaze is absent and sad. This does not appear to be a mere accident of photography.

Kolya leans jauntily on Anton's shoulder. His expression, alone among the faces, seems to show barely stifled levity. He is not so sturdy and handsome as his younger brother Anton. He is intriguing; but the photograph tells us little more about him. If we've learned elsewhere, already, about his artistic talent, his chaotic adult life and his early death, we try hard to read his appearance here.

Anton is a well-built boy, serious, and handsome. His features are regular. His gaze is clear. He has a fine forehead. We see, still, the roundness of his face and head that earned him the nickname "bomba," at school. Otherwise, the picture shows us only a fourteen-year-old still embedded in his large family.

How determinedly bourgeois the photograph is. And how patiently the family members have lent themselves to it. If film had been faster, in 1874, and the occasions for snapshots not so serious, a picture could tell us more about the family's relationships. This one, however, does have an interestingly dressed-up appearance. It is rather like Pavel's grocery store: the well fitted shop in front, with an upstairs drawing room for customers; but behind it, not visible from the street, the poor, crowded, dirty rooms in which the family lived, and which we've read about.

Here are several photographs from Anton's medical school days. In one picture of him in 1883, Anton Pavlovich still has the broad, stoic face that reminds us of his peasant origins. An oil painting of him by Kolya in 1894, however, emphasizes his good looks and his brooding intensity. He appears preoccupied, a little disheveled—one says at once, "a portrait of an artist." Of course, the artist Kolya made it, and did not emphasize the 'medical student'.

From Anton Pavlovich's university years, we find a photograph of Dr. Grigori Zakharin, Chekhov's favorite professor of medicine. More will be told in later chapters, of Dr. Zakharin's contribution to the shape of Chekhov's medical and literary careers. For now, we simply look at this grave, fine featured face. His eyes are sharply focused and considering. His intelligence is very clear. One cannot tell, really, what his profession might be; but vision, and single mindedness, must be part of it. To my eye, his face presents a contrast to Chekhov's. Both are surely thinkers. In most photographs, however, Anton Pavlovich looks more generally "afar," or inward. For all his love of science and objectivity, there is a hint here about Chekhov's need for his "mistress," literature. The "wife," medicine, when monogamously married, demands the kind of sharp focus we see so honed in Dr. Zakharin's features.

After graduation from medical school, and until his hospitalization for tuberculosis in 1897, Dr. A. P. Chekhov practiced medicine steadily. Photographs illuminate and animate this aspect of the writer's life. A prescription of Dr. Chekhov's is here reproduced. He orders zinc, and carbolic acid, for his patient. His writing is elegant, bold, legible , and well spaced. His signature, *Чеховъ*, sports that long, wavy tail that many of his correspondents and researchers have remarked on.

Here is a photograph of his stethoscope and reflex hammer: a dull picture, really, but useful history. This stethoscope is designed for one ear only. Looking like a small ear trumpet, it flowers to an open cone at one end, for placing on the patient's chest. Between the cone and the physician's earpiece is the straight metal listening tube, four or five inches long, which keeps the doctor's head just a bit apart from his patient. How symbolic of medicine this tool always is; and how much it changed in form over years. Anton Pavlovich's stethoscope gives us his historical placement.

Chekhov was photographed in the garden of his country estate at Melikhovo, in 1892. One of Russia's many cholera epidemics was erupting at the time. Dr. Chekhov was appointed to organize preparations for acute medical care in twenty-three villages of his home district. He stands before us in his overcoat and hat, just setting out for the day, probably, because he appears rested and alert. This time he looks us right in the eye; almost smiles. A fine, vigorous physician.

A picture from 1890, just before Chekhov's departure to interview prisoners in Sakhalin in Siberia, includes most of his family and several friends. They are sitting outside a house, on its steps. The picture is as commemorative as the family portrait of 1874, but is much less stiff. Better photographic techniques now allow this. And the change in seating arrangements is interesting. Now Anton sits front and center, and looks challengingly at us. Even his striped trousers and light-colored overcoat define him as different from the rest: the others are all dressed in dark suits and dresses. Pavel—moustache now as white as his beard—is in the back row, with his wife in front of him. He and Evgenia are somber. All the others are more cheerful.

In both these photographs, Anton Pavlovich shows vigor and engagement with the world. His leadership in the family, as well as the prospect of the medical adventure in Sakhalin, agree well with him, the 1890 photo attests. Professor Simon Karlinsky has chosen a picture of Chekhov from that same year, for inclusion as frontispiece for his 1973 book, *Letters of Anton Chekhov*. Here too, Anton Pavlovich looks youthful and well. (By now, we know however, he has had recurrent cough and blood-spitting for several years.) We see that Karlinsky has found a photograph that displays the Chekhov he himself admires: ". . . this supreme realist in life and in literature."[1] Here is a beautiful and intelligent face—which does not look straight at us, but a bit to the side, as if musing. Anton does not smile but is not gloomy. His hair, eyebrows and beard are well groomed. His lips are full and finely sculpted, in a face now more heart shaped than round. His peasant origin is no longer evident.

Anton Pavlovich chose his own preferred self-image, when he sent his photograph to Piotr Ilich Tchaikovsky in his late twenties. He was delighted and grateful, when the composer whose works he most admired called to express his admiration for Chekhov's work. The photograph is not unlike the one just described, with a similar pose. Anton Pavlovich's sartorial elegant simplicity shows a sensibility for this world. His facial expression is soft and spiritual; his eyes are focused to distance.

Images to see and names to sound give us, at least, a first introduction to a variety of Anton Pavlovic's close friends.

Anton met Isaak Levitan in 1879, when he began medical school. Levitan was then an art student comrade of Kolya's. He became a distinguished Russian landscape painter. The two men had in common their love of nature, and their similar approach to it in their different arts. They shared an appetite too for jokes, pranks and hoaxes. They were close friends for most of their lives—though estranged at times by their rivalry for women. Levitan often stayed at Chekhov's country estate, and frequently the two hunted together. Here is Levitan in 1890, dressed for serious hunting, gun under one arm, gun dog at his feet. He is extremely swarthy. His black eyebrows and thick beard have a weight oddly in contrast to his slenderness. He is already infected, we know, with the tuberculosis which will kill him ten years later. Levitan wounded a snipe, in 1892, while hunting with Chekhov. He begged his unwilling friend to kill it for him, and Anton at last did. Chekhov wrote to a friend later, "And while two idiots went home and sat down to dinner, there was one beautiful, enamored creature less in the world."[2] This incident, as well as a later "lovelorn" suicide attempt by Levitan with a loaded revolver, gave Chekhov images he used in *The Sea Gull* , which he was writing at the time.

Aleksei Suvorin was a major publisher and public figure in St. Petersburg. Chekhov was introduced to him in 1885. Shortly, Suvorin became Chekhov's chief publisher; then his close friend and most frequent correspondent for over a dozen years. The two men took many trips together, and often visited in each other's homes and families. There they talked for hours and hours—and continued the conversations in honest, intimate letters. Their similarities and differences somehow wove a strong attachment. Each man had a lowly beginning, a struggle for success, much loneliness and inner conflict in the process, and a fierce insistence on independence. Suvorin was born in Voronezh province, like Anton's father and grandfather. The two men understood each other. Also, we can suppose that as a boy, Anton experienced a great lack of practical help, affection, example, or steady care, from his father. Suvorin gave Anton all these things. And clearly, Suvorin relished giving them.

Pictures of these friends emphasize the twenty-year age gap between them, simply by photographing it. In an 1889 photo they stand together, smiling. These smiles have almost a family resemblance. Suvorin has developed a portliness, while Chekhov is youthfully slender. Then in a picture taken seven years later of Suvorin's family, with Anton Pavlovich, in a garden, Suvorin has aged considerably. His beard is now gray. He sits in an upstairs alcove flanked by two daughters, looking grandfatherly. Chekhov sits below among other Suvorin relatives—at ease, and centrally placed, as if a favorite son.

We may gather a bouquet of faces, each with its name, from among these portraits of women in Anton Pavlovich's life. In *Anton Chekhov, a Life*, Rayfield describes excellently what is known of them and their relations with Chekhov. Also, Carolina de Maegd-Soëp, in *Chekhov and Women in the Life and work of Chekhov, 1987*, discusses the impulses, ideals and constraints, which Anton Pavlovich brought to his love life. Here, the photographs alone are illuminating.

Chekhov said that beauty was his primary requirement in a woman. He also made other—often contradictory—pronouncements. The "true nature" of women seemed always to puzzle and worry him. In his student days, he thought seriously of writing a doctoral thesis on the *History of Sexual*

Authority. Were females born inferior to males? From extensive reading (and with scientific detachment!), Anton Pavlovich deduced that the higher the social development was in the various mammals, the more nearly equal the sexes became. He remained convinced however, of the inferiority of even the most educated female human being. These pictures of some of his loves show us the range of his more personal exploration, before he married Olga Knipper in 1901.

Here is Lika Mizinova. Her photograph from 1890 shows us her striking appearance: long rippling blonde hair, heavy dark eyebrows over soft, lighter eyes; and a lovely full mouth. No wonder Masha described her nineteen-year-old friend Lika like this: "People could not take their eyes off her. My girlfriends often stopped me and asked, 'Chekhova, tell me, who is that beauty with you'."[3] Lika, like Masha, was studying to be a teacher. But she yearned to be an actress. She fell in love with Anton, for life. And sometimes, he loved her.

A contrast is Natalia Golden, whom Anton also met when he was twenty-one. Unlike her voluptuous sister Anna—both of them in this 1883 photograph—Natalia is slender, and dark, with an aquiline nose and a brooding expression. Anton called her "Natashevu" (Natash-chez-vous). He stayed many of his medical school nights with her.

And Olga Kundasova is here, with her questioning, piercing eyes, a very slight smile, a very plain hairdo with a midline part like George Eliot's. She was an astronomer at the Moscow Observatory; a sometime lover of Anton's who came and went tumultuously in his life until the time of his funeral.

Elena Shavrova, the youngest of the Shavrova 'three sisters', is photographed at age twenty. At fifteen, she was a budding writer who dared to approach Chekhov in a cafe to ask for advice on a story. Anton mentored her, rejected her, made love to her, at various times over the years. Here she appears as a well-coiffed young blonde lady. Not much is discernable beyond the prosperousness of her elegant dress. She is pretty, but not beautiful.

The name of the actress Kleopatra Karatygina is attractive indeed. She is, however, in this photograph, neither beautiful nor happy-looking. She was one of the group of actresses in Moscow with whom Anton Pavlovich spent time in 1889. After the death of his brother Kolya, Chekhov was bitter and depressed for many months; alternately, he sought escape and distraction. He visited the actresses he met in connection with production of his plays—relaxed with them and was doted upon. Kleopatra fell in love with him. There was a brief sexual affair, but no ongoing intimacy. Others among the actresses who "adored" Chekhov were more sensuous, histrionic, calculating and playful. In an 1893 photograph that its subjects called "The Temptations of St. Anthony," Tatiana Shchepkina-Kupernik and Lidia Iavorskaia sit turned towards Anton with rapturous faces. Lidia, a beautiful and elegant blonde, stretches out her arm towards him. Anton Pavlovich sits with rather smug satisfaction in his chair, looking at the photographer rather than the ladies.

Professor Rayfield chose I.E. Braz' portrait of Chekhov in 1898, for reproduction on his book jacket. This was indeed the 'official portrait' of Chekhov in his later years of great fame and declining health. Anton's artist friend Levitan had urged that Braz be commissioned for the task, since Braz was the outstanding Russian portrait painter of the time. The picture was hung the next year in the important Tretyakov Gallery in Moscow. Braz had joined Chekhov's family at their country estate in Melikhovo to paint it. Then he followed Chekhov to Nice to redo it. For all this, Anton and his family disliked the painting heartily. Anton ". . . loathed the Jeremiah-like expression which Braz had captured so well."[4] And there is more that may have pained him. Anton Pavlovich appears in the portrait as a middle-aged man in poor health. Can he be only thirty-eight? He leans his cheek against his left hand as though needing this support. The skin of his hands and face has pale, or greenish, undertones; while his nose is reddened. And though his clothing is more richly elegant than in the earlier photographs, and the pince-nez bespeaks gravity and learning, his sorrowful eyes quite undo any image of contented success.

Finally, we may study one enlarged photograph of Anton Pavlovich and his wife Olga. This fills a whole page of Dr. Coope's book on Chekhov. Its effect is immediate and poignant. Chekhov's big black coat is the largest mass in the image—but his smile and that of Olga, who leans her chin on his shoulder and presses against him, easily captures the focus of the picture. Anton's beard is pepper-and-salt. His hair is tousled. The pince-nez is in place, but a little askew, so it does not hide his happy eyes. Olga's eyes too are joyful. She is a very pretty woman, lively and responsive-looking. Olga is a Moscow actress of German family, who stars in Anton Pavlovich's plays. She is eight years younger than he. Here, the age difference appears even more. But their harmonious fit is plain.

In one other photo, Chekhov is standing in his Yalta garden with two of his dogs. There is the familiar big black overcoat, black trousers and shoes and hat. An older man's costume. The grizzly beard, pince-nez, and the cane he is carrying, add to the aged impression. Anton Pavlovich's face bears creases and wrinkles. He is looking down at a dog, with a half smile.

These dogs of his are small and crookedy, not very handsome. One is white, one black. Both regard the photographer intently. The nearer dog cocks his head a little. He has one white paw, on an otherwise all-black body. One imagines Chekhov noticing this from time to time and being amused. Or he is amused, and bemused, at where he finds himself in these final years.

III.
A Medical Career

Chekhov was a practicing physician. A picture forms in our minds of his professional behavior and habits of mind, as like our own doctors'. But his medical work was combined with an exceptional literary career. This in turn unexpectedly influenced his ways of doctoring. And just as important, the role of physician was in transition, in Russia, at the time Anton Pavlovich began his medical training. If we in the West wonder about his choice of this career, his experiences and vicissitudes, we must pay attention to this.

Ten years or less before Anton's birth, a Russian doctor could expect little honor or status. His medical school education had featured many stale lectures, and very little practical experience. He could offer his patients only palliation, since the causes of diseases and the action of medicaments were not yet understood. He had no social prestige and very poor earning power. Aristocrats might consult him, but treated him as a servant. Peasants were suspicious of him and kept to their own notions of treatment.

At mid-century, however, a wind of change blew from the West. Pasteur, and Lister, and Koch, had established a new germ theory of diseases. Antisepsis, permitting healing and safe surgery, could now be practiced. Cures were truly possible. In Russia, the field of medicine, like most vocations, remained under strict regulation by the Tsar's government. The Tsar wished, however, to bring the country's medicine up to wider world standards. The curriculum and level of teaching at the Moscow Medical Faculty was upgraded. I can attest that these improvements, and the ideals and teaching methods of Anton's best professors in the 1880's, still set a standard in my own medical school days at Johns Hopkins

School of Medicine in the 1940's. Some of his professors were seminal scientists whose work we studied.

Dr. Dubrowski, the Tsar's own physician, became Director of the Medical-Surgical Academy. He had both administrative skills and power to make rapid improvements. More government scholarships were now offered to poor but promising medical student applicants, so that the country's pool of doctors might improve and enlarge. Anton Chekhov secured one of these scholarships, $300/year, from the Taganrog city council. Whatever his motives for deciding on this career—he himself said, "I do not remember exactly what prompted me to choose medical school, but I have no reason to regret the choice"[1]—Anton Pavlovich must have seen that there was a reasonable livelihood to be had in this now quite hopeful field.

In the first year of the improved five-year curriculum in Moscow, students studied anatomy, chemistry and other laboratory subjects. They then progressed to observing patients with their professors; and finally to treating them, under supervision. The professors' lectures were outstanding in Chekhov's time. Aleksandr Babukhin was a gifted speaker on histology: he is most probably Chekhov's inspiration for Professor Stepanovich in "A Dreary Story." Eric Erismann, a Swiss-born professor of public health, talked passionately about the social issues of poverty and poor working conditions as matters most relevant to Russian health. For Anton Pavlovich, the lectures of Grigori Zakharin, Professor of Medicine, were most excellent. Zakharin emphasized the importance to a doctor of detailed history taking. This must include the patient's life style, and his psychological state. He once devoted eight successive lectures to the description of a single patient, a tailor from Moscow with chronic abdominal pain. He also, like Erismann, dwelt on public health issues of poverty, malnutrition, pollution. Long after graduation,

Chekhov sometimes returned to the university to listen to Zakharin.

There were stiff examinations for graduation, at the end of five years. The student was then certified as a "lekar," or general practitioner. He was eligible to practice—and also was exempted from military service, and from the Russian poll tax. He could earn the postgraduate degree of "M.D." by submitting a presentable thesis. If he hoped to teach at the university, this was required.

What then? The next choice of the young doctor lay between practice in the public sector, "zemstvo medicine" as will be described; getting a hospital position as aide and student to some outstanding specialist (such positions were few); or private practice in the city or provinces. Postgraduate internships and residencies have long been considered an essential last step in a doctor's training, in the West. This was not at all supported by the Tsarist government—which set the rules, and took no advice from practicing physicians themselves.

Zemstvos were district government organizations set up across Russia by Tsar Nicholas I, then strengthened by Alexander II in 1864 in his "great reforms." All classes of citizens were eligible for election to zemstvo posts. While operating money, and most important decisions, continued to be issued by the Tsar's central ministries in St. Petersburg, there was at least a measure of local self-government. Hospitals, clinics and public health matters were among the zemstvos' departments. Moscow province had a particularly progressive zemstvo. There, health education for citizens was provided as well as treatment. Research was done on the correlation of disease with geographical and environmental factors. Dr. Erismann, for example, surveyed the condition of factory workers in Moscow. For his political activities, he was dismissed from his professorship in 1896.

Three quarters of Russia's doctors went to work for zemstvos, in Chekhov's day. Many did this, in cities and villages, for idealistic reasons. Here was a program promising free health care to all citizens in a time of great oppression and poverty in Russia. Also, young doctors needed the regular salary, meager as it was. Those poor medical students who had received government stipends had to repay them in two to ten years. Few general practitioners could live or support families on fees collected in private practice. Neither peasants in the villages nor the average city dwellers could afford much. Only a very few doctors had the social connections for a lucrative city practice, or hope for a professorship.

The central government enforced strict rules for physicians. They must answer any call for medical help, at any time, or be prosecuted. They must perform their share of autopsies; also work for the zemstvo in times of epidemic or famine. If Jewish, they were not eligible for any salaried position. Thirty-seven percent of all doctors died of infectious diseases. Their suicides accounted for ten percent of the country's annual suicides in the 25-35-year age range. And there was no government health or retirement fund for zemstvo physicians.

A general practitioner like Dr. Chekhov saw every sort of human malady. He would treat for broken bones, broken sleep, headache, heart attack, stroke, carbuncles, childbirth with complications, failure of the liver or kidneys, erysipelas, tuberculosis: that is only a beginning. If poor diet or industrial pollution was a prime factor in his patient's illness, there was little he could do about it. Most taxing and tragic were the epidemic waves of deadly diseases like cholera, typhus, typhoid, which swept regularly over large regions. Here, the discoveries of Lister and Koch had begun to make a real difference. When Dr. Chekhov headed a program to contain cholera in his district in 1892, he was of the first generation that knew how sanitation, disinfection, also the hydration and isolation of the actively ill, could lower the death rate dramatically. The education of the peasant patients who distrusted all this—they sometimes saw "killers" in the doctors arriving at their villages—was a slower process. As to available medicaments in general: one learns from Chekhov, and from other doctors' memoirs, that drugs might indeed alleviate painful symptoms, but could not alter the basic course of the diseases. Typical prescriptions were for calomel, castor oil, potassium iodide, salicylates, napthalene, valerian, arsenic, creosote.

A last item of background to Anton Pavlovich's medical career is political turmoil. Over the years of his practice, doctors were swept up in a rising protest to the Tsar's rule. Yet as Nancy Frieden says in *Russian Physicians in an Era of Reform and Revolution, 1856-1905*, "Only a small segment of the profession allied itself with the radical intelligentsia. By training and necessity physicians are pragmatists . . . forced to compromise in daily tasks. In medicine the answers are rarely definitive or final."[2] This was indeed Chekhov's stance, for both professional and personal reasons. In medical school he was seen attending student protest meetings, but did not actively participate. On the inflaming issues, such as the obstacles to women's education, and the degradation of Jews, he spoke out in his own circle, and personally helped female and Jewish friends. But once, he wrote of a poet's inspiring political song of the times, "Forward without Fear or Doubt," "If you cry 'Forward!', you must without fail explain in which direction one must go. Do you not see that, if, without explaining the direction, you fire off this word simultaneously at a monk and at a revolutionary, they will proceed in precisely opposite directions?"[3] Chekhov did not work for a zemstvo except in times of epidemic, as will be discussed. But he wrote in an 1890 letter, ". . . if I were offered a choice between the 'ideals' of the celebrated sixties and today's poorest zemstvo hospital, I'd take the latter without the least hesitation."[4] In the literary field, he took a very public political stand in resigning from the Academy of Sciences when Maksim Gorki, newly elected, was promptly expelled by order of the Tsar's government. Even this, in support of his friend, he did rather slowly and reluctantly; always distrustful of easy gestures.

Meanwhile during Chekhov's adult life, there was a steady pressure towards professional autonomy and political influence by doctors. Even before Anton's birth, a famous medical scientist, Dr. Grigor Pirogov, had so abhorred the medical conditions of the army and the Russian populace during the Crimean War that he poured his energy and influence into reforms. Through the progressive zemstvos, and a "Pirogov Society" of physicians, he influenced a whole generation of doctors to distrust bureaucratic control, to champion the careers of women and of Jews, and to fight for an independent 'guild' of doctors on the Western model, setting its own standards of practice and education. Not unexpectedly, in 1866 he drew government fire and was forced to resign. Dr. Zakharin, Chekhov's hero, lost his professorship too when in 1894 he was falsely accused of poisoning Tsar Alexander III in his last illness. These were severe setbacks. However, in the late decades of the century, doctors won skirmishes against the bureaucrats, with the power that being indispensable during epidemics and famines gave them. The government counterattacked as soon as was expedient. It planned to write a "Hospital Statute" which would take back considerable control of medical practice from the zemstvo physicians. Zemstvo opposition and the Pirogov Society succeeded in forcing indefinite postponement of the plan. The Pirogov Society took on more and more social issues. By 1902, it fought (unsuccessfully) against corporal punishment of citizens, against the state's liquor monopoly, etc. At the 9th Pirogov Congress in 1904—the year of Chekhov's death—2,136 physicians attended, as well as thousands of medical students, paramedics, and citizens. It was declared that the usual petitions to the government were now useless. There must be direct action. And in 1905, many doctors joined in the first Russian Revolution.

A certain "Dr. V. Veresaeff"—a pseudonym for Dr. V. Sindovich—wrote a serialized article in the magazine *Mir Boji* in 1901. This was published as a book, *The Confessions of a Physician*, in a London edition of 1904. Against the historical background just presented, I would like to describe this physician's experience. His book was important at the time in raising his colleagues' political consciousness. It divided those who read it into "Veresaevites" and "Antiveresaevites." The educated public was shocked at the state of Russian medicine, which V. depicted. It is said that many young people, on reading the book, decided they would not become doctors. Even the American editor of the Knopf edition, a few years later, felt he must justify in his introduction the publishing of so "unsettling" a book.

My chief reason for presenting Veresaeff to you is that he serves as both corroborator and contrast to Anton Chekhov's career. Here are two men who followed the paths of education and medical practice in Russia at about the same time. Veresaeff was only seven years out of Moscow University Medical School when he wrote his book; he graduated ten years after Chekhov did so from that same school. I know of him only what he tells us here. One obvious fact is that he was not, like Chekhov, a highly skilled writer. He was, however, sensitive, passionate, and frank enough to impress the educated readers of his time. He set himself to tell his countrymen the truth about his experiences.

V. says he was a good but rather casual scholar at his gymnasia. "The advance of my mental development was quite independent of my school, and it was outside school hours that I accumulated the knowledge of those facts which interested me."[5] This, like Anton Pavlovich. He assessed himself as "average" in intelligence and skills. On entering medical school, he was entranced by the theories of the natural sciences. He soon accustomed himself to the shock of dissecting a human corpse, for anatomy. Science was supreme, he felt, "[it could make] all deviation from its straight path a sheer impossibility."[6]

His clinical years in medical school were unexpectedly miserable, however. He was anguished by the sufferings of patients. He had not yet received training in their treatment, but he did have to diagnose them in front of professors and colleagues. He often failed at this. Sometimes the professor then took over and demonstrated to his shame how simple the diagnosis really was. But on occasion, Veresaeff observed his medical teacher making a misdiagnosis. This was never corrected—in fact, any later lethal effects of it were well hidden. Professors in the various specialties colluded in this. The families of dying patients never suspected. V. was tormented by ethical questions. How could the poor, in the clinics, be used so cavalierly as 'demonstrations' for medical students? How could women be shamed this way by naked exhibition—and were he and his colleagues lecherous in watching? How could autopsies be required, when the dissection of their loved one meant only desecration to the bereaved families?

Veresaeff passed his final examinations, by reading ten to twelve hours a day in the last months. He crammed into his head information which he considered three-fourths "ballast." He had to plan for the narrow self-interest of each examining professor: ". . . most important of all was to know the individual hobbies and foibles of the examiner."[7] Still, he hoped to digest his training as he opened his practice. "Later on, when I have more leisure, I will think it all over and put everything straight."[8]

He hung out his shingle very unready. (He decided not to work for a zemstvo, because the salary there would not support him and his family.) Veresaeff looked "with bitter envy" on those few classmates who got house-physician jobs, as Anton Pavlovich had done in his day, and thus got some hands-on training. His first patients terrified him. He had no actual experience of the effects of the available medications; nor did he know how they actually worked. He lanced abscesses and removed patients' growths, but had never before held a scalpel in his hand. It is painful to read of V's early mistakes, some of them lethal, though never intentional. No wonder he usually had difficulty in accepting payment.

Veresaeff decided he must have more supervised training, and left private practice. He found no openings on the paid house staff of St. Petersburg hospitals; so became a 'supernumerary' doctor in one, with no pay whatever. There he did gain experience. But he received no meals, and says he managed to subsist solely on vodka for awhile. Then he returned to private practice. Eventually he obtained a hospital appointment too, at seventy-five rubles a month. Somehow he supported himself, his wife, and two children.

The hit-or-miss basis of medication continued to trouble him. Turning to the medical journals, he at first was reassured by their detailed analyses—but began to notice the fads, the swift reversals of opinions on each drug, while meanwhile many patients had been damaged. He himself caused the death of some patients by prescribing on this "excellent advice." "A catastrophe may overwhelm you at any moment and ruin you for life,"[9] he said.

He found solace in doing some scientific experimental work. "[There] one had no need to grope about in obscurity; it was possible to institute complete control over one's every step."[10] This sensitive man was appalled, however, by the pain and death inflicted on living animals. For him it was another dilemma in medicine. Knowledge must be expanded. Callous experiment on trusting patients must be stopped. But vivisection too harms living creatures.

Veresaeff concluded that the medical profession was a dubious one. Learning and experience may somewhat help; but practice is unfortunately an art, and this young man, though reasonably intelligent and very dedicated, despaired about his own creativity. Confidence and love may be offered to the "godlike doctor" by patients. But the doctor is a sham—and is required to be. The profession itself is unjust. Jewish doctors practice under slavish conditions. Women are maltreated both as patients and as colleagues. Doctors generally are overworked, underpaid: they commit suicide, or drink, or die young of exhaustion.

His thoughts were turning more and more to his discovery that poverty and ignorance were the basic causes of most illnesses. ". . . A physician must first of all strive to remove those conditions which at present render his work both senseless and barren . . . he must be a public worker in the broadest sense of the term."[11] Too many doctors were self-righteous and exploiting, he said. "It is time [for change], high time!"[12]

No wonder that V.'s voice rallied many of his peers, and the students, to be activists for political change in the profession and the country. I could find no evidence of Chekhov's reading or commenting on Veresaeff's book. But Anton Pavlovich's words to a neighboring doctor, in the late 1890's, raised a similar issue indeed. "It is time that zemstvo doctors and other medical workers stopped turning up their noses at the press. They should all join in newspaper controversies in their areas, especially the public health doctors who refuse to do this out of pride."[13]

Anton Pavlovich told his intimate friends, in letters, about experiencing many of the injustices and disillusions that Veresaeff describes. These appear in his stories and plays as well. Dr. Astrov in *Uncle Vanya* describes them vividly. "On my feet from morning to night with never a moment's peace, and then lying under the bedclothes afraid of being dragged out to a patient", he tells the old nurse. A patient under his care died in surgery: "And just when I least wanted it my feelings seemed to wake up again, and my conscience began to worry me as if I had killed him deliberately."[14] This could be Veresaeff, or Chekhov, speaking. These men spoke directly for themselves, however. Let us look at Anton Pavlovich's own journey through his career in that light.

He came to Moscow University with a good gymnasia education, but no particular studious bent. His first encounter with scientific rigor and aims fired him at once. He aimed at objectivity, careful proof, for the rest of his medical career; and by his own words, kept a similar standard in his writing. Dr. Zakharin and other mentors truly influenced his life.

Anton Palvovich was never a drudge. Making new friends, male and female—drinking, joking, visiting the theater and the brothels—filled much of his time when he was not at home dealing with the family, or dashing off short stories for magazines. He showed typical medical student pride and superiority in his new knowledge. He offered it frequently to his family and friends; meanwhile complaining to others of these "demands" on a young doctor. He earned only an average mark in his anatomy study. But his fellow student, Grigori Rossolimo, noticed that Anton read unusually widely in non-required texts. Darwin, and Claude Bernard, for example, were just then published. Anton made notes for his own scientific inquiry into *A History of Sexual Authority* in human beings—which he never finished.

Rossolimo described Chekhov as very shy, almost unnoticeable, at school. As the clinical studies began, however, he often stood out for his ease and excellence at interviewing patients. Dr. Pavel Arkhangelsky also remarked on this. Chekhov worked under Dr. Arkhangelsky in the

Chikino Hospital at Voskresensk in the last summers of his medical school training. This mentor noticed Anton Pavlovich's sometimes hesitant manner, at his tasks; but also how attentive and kind he was to his patients, and how much their mental state interested him. The two men became friends. Anton Pavlovich was invited after graduation to work awhile at Chikino, and then briefly at the nearby Zvenigorod Hospital. He had a frightening experience there, as a novice—much as Veresaeff describes his own. Anton Pavlovich could not manage the necessary manipulations, in an emergency operation on a five-year-old boy, and had to call for help from a local doctor. He felt more competent however, even exhilarated, at doing medico-legal investigations and autopsies. Then in the fall he returned to Moscow, and opened a private practice.

We can identify some traits in Chekhov, which saved him from the severe miseries and doubts which young V. endured.

First, certainly, was his high intelligence, of a steady and adaptable kind. He seemed able to retain dry information as required—just enough of it—and to have wits left over for his own thoughts and projects.

Crowded and hectic as his family life was, it probably gave him ballast. Anton was truly important to his siblings, respected by his parents, and he was the principal breadwinner. He had to take time from his books to write fiction; luckily for us all.

Anton Pavlovich had firsthand knowledge from childhood of the physical and psychological effects of poverty and abuse. Medical school cannot provide this. He had lived among both peasants and the upper classes. He knew ladies, and whores. A young man who had played in cemeteries, who'd mistreated some animals as a boy, who could mimic the hypocrisies of bureaucrats and of his father, could keep afloat in those medical school situations, which so appalled tender Veresaeff. It was crucial to his development that Chekhov could wholeheartedly admire a few of his professors. Luckily, he already knew that leaders may have feet of clay, and was not shaken. He may have deplored the use of female clinic patients for demonstration—but I doubt that he "blushed" at the sight.

Chekhov rarely exposed his fears and doubts to others, in any connection. The giving of dubious or useless medicines to patients did not seem to trouble him. As a medical student he relished his new power to do this. To Aleksandr, for example, he wrote an "authoritative recommendation" of "decoct salep or an *otvar* of althea, both with a drop of opium", to be given to his brother's baby for diarrhea. "I don't want to improvise . . . It will all be based on the latest scientific evidence."[15] He was still enthusiastic about the pharmacopoeia at age thirty-six, when he wrote to Suvorin about his medical plans to fight cholera in the villages. A skeptical attitude towards "cures" is evident in letters to various friends he treated. But in my own reading about Dr. Chekhov, I am impressed with the level-headed expertise he gradually developed. He made competent use of medicaments though they had considerable limits.

Anton Pavlovich's personality, finally, helped him get a solid education. He was poor. He had no doctors in his family, nor useful connections. Yet Dr. Arkhangelsky invited him to a modestly paid position in his hospital after graduation, even though Chekhov was still a rather uncertain practitioner. (How Veresaeff had wished for that!) Some fellow classmates like Rossolimo remained helpful, lifelong friends; though they'd become "one career" outstanding doctors, and he a "dual career" practitioner.

Sometimes, both in medicine and in literature, Chekhov used his charm consciously. Sometimes he acknowledged that to friends; but did not agonize about it. When he received the Pushkin Prize for his literary work when he was only twenty-six, he'd been energetically sponsored by the famous writer

Grigorovich, and the influential editor Suvorin. He wondered if he'd deceived the judges "just as I deceive many people with my face".[16] That may be a questionable ability. Most of us, still, want our doctor to have it.

Chekhov's literary career has been studied more widely than his medical life. I would like here to follow the latter, briefly, from start to finish. His literary life so flowered that it often took precedence. His practice sometimes lapsed for this reason—and more and more because of illness. Consumption, finally, took his shingle down from the door. Yet he grew professionally; played an honorable role in his consulting room, and was generous of his time and effort to the zemstvo.

After the first summer at Voskresensk and Zvenigorod hospitals, Anton Pavlovich set up practice in his Moscow house. Patients were slow to appear, and when they did, paid poorly. Most were friends and family. He augmented his income by performing autopsies, and by medical work in the Moscow brothels. Between patients with rashes, toothaches, dysentery, etc., he had scraps of time to write his short stories for the magazines. Two bad moments for this new practitioner are recorded. Once, he realized he'd made a mistake on a prescription—and rushed into the street to chase the departing patient in a rental carriage, to retrieve it. The other was a more serious moment. A pleasant family, the Ianovs, were his patients and friends. When the mother and three daughters fell ill of typhoid, he could not save the mother and one daughter. He was so shaken that he told his brother he might give up medicine entirely. He did, however, continue to practice, and the two surviving sisters remained his friends.

Chekhov rented a house in the country near Voskresensk, the next summer, for his family. There at Babkino he doctored nearby peasants, neighbors, friends and family. Rickets, rashes, accidents, were among these poor peasants' ailments. When two years later he was able to rent a summer estate near

Sumy in the Ukraine, he was relieved that the Ukrainian peasants were more "civilized," less "diseased and degraded," so he could sometimes "forget he was a doctor"[17] and do more writing there. Chekhov's landlord and his three daughters became his friends. Anton Pavlovich helped the middle daughter, who was physician for this area, with her surgery and treatments. It is plain from his description of this that he was more sure of himself medically, by now—and that he enjoyed buoying up his good but timid colleague. "I bear glad tidings where she sees death; and I double the doses she prescribes."[18] When the patient must inevitably die, Anton tried to cheer up this anguished woman doctor.

In the letters, Chekhov's doctoring of friends and family is frequently mentioned. He examined and prescribed for many literary friends who visited from Moscow and St. Petersburg. The elderly writer Grigorovich, the famous old poet Pleshcheev, were under his care; and the editors Leiken and Suvorin. He brought his sick friend Levitan to his house, and his dying brother Kolya. Both men were difficult, at times impossible, patients. Levitan had periods of paranoid psychosis. Kolya, dying of tuberculosis, was also increasingly sick in his frantic, dishonest and exploitative behavior. This cost Kolya his artistic career, and many friendships. Both men would beg Anton Pavlovich to treat them, then leave his house without warning and return to chaotic lives, as soon as they were physically able.

I have wondered—as a present day, Western, urban physician—at Chekhov's readiness to act as doctor to intimate friends and family. Doctors today are discouraged from doing this, if at all possible. The reasons are clear. Medical judgment can be twisted by intense personal feeling for the patient. And the responsibility for these patients' misery, pain and possible death is a heavy burden. In treating Kolya, Anton suffered and sometimes faltered. His circumstances were of the time, however. The family and friends, perhaps, could not have found other doctors they trusted. Many of them were poor and asked for Chekhov's free care. Whatever the reasons—we do see in his experiences why the caveat has been more recently imposed.

Kolya's death , at Anton's home and under Anton's care, of a disease which was active in his own lungs, was profoundly unsettling. Chekhov reacted with restlessness and irritability during the next few months. His medical work was interrupted by his many trips; and at the same time he expressed strong revulsion for his "mistress," literature. Writing was a shoddy business. He thought himself a shoddy writer, too. Chekhov salvaged his dwindling self esteem, six months after Kolya's death, by a sudden decision to visit the Island of Sakhalin as a doctor. His wife, medicine, would restore him—in this case through the rigors of a hard journey, and a months' long piece of work, reporting objectively on all he found at the Russian penal colony. He hoped for real social impact, from the book he would write on Sakhalin's grim conditions. He also hoped his book would be accepted at Moscow University as his long overdue thesis for the M.D. degree. He would feel he had "[paid] off some of my debt to medicine, towards which, as you know, I've behaved like a pig."[19] Also, he would then be eligible to teach. Dr. Rossolimo had long invited him to give a special course for students, in which Chekhov would invite them to understand what illness really feels like, and encourage them to identify with many kinds of patients. Such an academic role would be dear to Anton Pavlovich.

His book was not accepted as a thesis. On return from his journey, however, and after a period of illness, and travel, he remained faithful to medicine. He bought an estate for himself and his family in the village of Melikhovo, fifty miles south of Moscow. There he set up at once to practice medicine.

Anton enlisted his younger brother Ivan to bring medical supplies from Moscow, and his sister Masha to help him again as surgical nurse, pharmacist, and office manager. A nurse assistant was later employed too. His brother Mikhail later described the flow of peasant patients who visited Anton, "from 25 to 50 versts away" every day, with a wide assortment of maladies.[20] Chekhov footed the bill for medicines and supplies. The peasants paid him largely in animals and goods. The doctor made house calls on demand, in horse and carriage, to the point of exhaustion.

Chekhov had learned in medical school that sanitation, and nutrition, are most important in containing disease. He used this knowledge when he organized medical responses to cholera epidemics in the 1890's. He personally arranged for medical supplies for his villages, found room for hospital beds, rounded up staff. He canvassed wealthy landowners in the region for financial aid and for the loan of their rooms for hospital care. Many of these nobles refused. The lowly doctor was treated cavalierly. Such humiliation is described by Veresaeff; and by V.F. Snegirev thus, in his eulogy for Dr. Zakharin in 1896. "Who can forget how the doctor once stood in the doorway afraid to take a seat? How some doctors were only allowed to treat peasants, and others appeared like a watch maker in a frockcoat at an established hour to ask about the health of the master of the household."[21] Anton Pavlovich complained about the selfish gentry in letters to friends. But he was in general exhilarated by his work preparing for cholera. He was pleased by the treatment regime he devised for his villages. ". . . The enemas have a wonderful effect . . . the injections sometimes produce miracles."[22] And to Suvorin he wrote, "I was wild with rapture on reading about the cholera . . . it is a pity that you aren't a physician and cannot share my satisfaction; that is to say truly feel and realize and understand all that is being done."[23]

Dr. Chekhov also had his fatigue, boredom, and even disgust. "A doctor has terrible days and hours"[24], he wrote to Suvorin. His sister Masha has described his steadfast availability to all calls for help. "He sometimes frowned when they came for him when he was ill or very tired. But once we helped our brother to dress his frown disappeared and the man waiting on the porch could not see any sign of discontent on his face."[25] Beyond Melikhovo, he gave many individuals health advice, or money. He raised funds to save the prestigious journal, *The Surgical Chronicle,* from demise, because the whole profession depended on it. Meanwhile, his worsening tuberculosis brought him fevers, fatigue and hemorrhages. And he was writing, at Melikhovo: "The Grasshopper," "Ward Six," *The Island of Sakhalin*, "Big Volodia and Little Volodia," "The Black Monk," "Three Years," "Ariadne," "The House with the Mezzanine," "My Life"—and *The Seagull.* Productions of his plays, as well as social life and general restlessness, often took him to Moscow or St. Petersburg for weeks at a time. When home, however, he resumed his practice.

Anton's sudden hospitalization, at age thirty-seven, marked the end of his medical practice. He never again held office hours or answered to emergencies. He still prescribed and diagnosed for certain friends, and family, and for new acquaintances in Nice and Yalta where he himself was ill. He nursed his wife Olga after her operation for ectopic pregnancy—but could manage that only briefly, because it so exhausted him.

He would die only two years later. Still, he continued his commitment to social medicine. He raised funds for a sanatorium for the many indigent consumptives who came to Yalta. He sent books and money for schools in Taganrog, Melikhovo and other provincial towns. In his letters, Chekhov sometimes complained to his friends about the burden of all this. He was an affluent and famous man who was very often petitioned. However, he had sought out many of these causes. Chekhov followed in the path of the teachers he honored—Zakharin, and Erismann—keeping a wide view of proper work for a Russian physician. He also had powerful personal standards.

It is surprising to discover what Anton P. Chekhov was doing, through the years of his greatest writing. He compiled an entire census, door to door, on the Island of Sakhalin. He visited starving villages in Nizhni Novgorod, to report on them "objectively." He never stopped sitting on committees, working as a fund raiser; and even ran a bazaar one day with his sister. Was he spendthrift with his precious time? The sixteen-year-old Anton must be remembered. He was left alone in Taganrog, without the family, to scrounge a living. He must finish school, fend off father's creditors, send money to his mother in Moscow. He did all this, and somehow found ample time for his own vivid experiences. The pattern held throughout his life—somehow a matter of balancing, and sometimes very intricate. Chekhov's balance, in fact, deserves its own chapter.

IV.
A Particular Balance

Were we determined to "understand" Nijinsky's great art—only the secret of his dancing style, that is, not even to approach the personal story from which he created it—we would not succeed. We watch the grainy early films, and agree on the astounding levitation of his leaps. In transitions from one physical action to another, however difficult, he keeps unwavering poise. He has pyrotechnic balance. Knowledge of the length of his femur would not explain it for us. Talking with him about his intents or his sensations in leaping would have fascinated us, but that is not quite "understanding."

I think that Anton Chekhov's resources for personal equilibrium were as rich as Nijinsky's for dancing. His balancing techniques were complicated, and often hidden even from himself. This may account for the hard time biographers have had, to present Chekhov whole. It was, however, what allowed him to live and to create, despite illness, to the age of forty-four. I have not understood it all, either. What follows is a gathering of instances of his keeping the balance. They come from his life events, his contemporaries' view of him, his own letters, and sometimes from lines of his stories and plays.

It can be said that the boy Anton Pavlovich was an abused child. In the spirit of Chekhov, let us replace that overused phrase with simple evidence of it.

Pavel Egorovich, Anton's father, was by most accounts a man who patterned his parenting after his own father's. Egor beat his sons frequently for "any misdemeanor—picking apples, or falling off a roof they were making. Pavel developed a hernia after one punishment, and had to wear a truss for it throughout his adult life."[1] Egor insisted on education for his sons; but did not match this concern with any signs of affection. He was a bully: his farm workers called him "the viper." On paper he could be rhetorical, obfuscating, or sentimental. All this is equally true of his son, Pavel. The wives of both father and son were beaten down and depressed, not able to act as counterforce for their children against the father's overbearing.

Some biographers and critics have described Pavel as simply typical of Russian lower class fathers at the time. Poor men's children had to be molded into acceptable, employable adults by whatever methods. Meanwhile, their role was to help and obey parents. Pavel earns credit for his dogged insistence that his sons be educated. Also, because of his own love of church music and his religiosity, he exposed the children to large doses of both. They all became openly irreligious as soon as possible—still, Anton could find a deep love of music, and a spirituality in himself, in spite of Pavel's skewed presentation. But we note that the thrashings Pavel inflicted on his three oldest children were heavier and more frequent than the norm of their extended family or of other Taganrog households. The adult Anton told a friend, "You know, my father thrashed me so much when I was a child that I still cannot forget it."[2] Aleksandr wrote, "It was a sheer Tatar yoke, without a glimmer of light . . . I look back on my childhood with crushing anguish."[3] A grade school chum of Anton's who sometimes visited the house remembered, "in the Chekhov household . . . as soon as his father appeared we went quiet and ran home. He had a heavy hand. He punished children for the most innocent naughtiness . . ."[4]

This is physical abuse. And for the Chekhov children, other aspects of their father were equally damaging and oppressive. Anton once wrote to Aleksandr, "tyranny and lies crippled our childhood so much that it makes me sick and afraid to remember. Remember the horror and revulsion we felt in those days when father would flare up because the soup was over-salted, or would curse mother for a fool."[5] Pavel supervised all aspects of his children's behavior by posting a "roster" of their daily duties at home. Those found wanting would be punished. When they were away from home, his letters in the same vein would follow. He invoked the word of God frequently to back up his dictums. As Anton remarked, there was no forgiveness in this version of the Deity. Nor did Pavel show interest in the individual natures or talents of his children, except as they needed correction. Most remarkable was Pavel's seeming lack of self awareness. He left Taganrog for Moscow because of his business collapse; yet badgered his 16-year-old son Anton in letters to hurry up and send money, appease creditors, as if he himself were not responsible. He aimed well at arousing guilt in Anton by describing "mother's tears." Anton's letters to his cousin Misha at the time show his love for his mother, as well as his sense of her fragility. "Half moribund"[6], he called her. For her part, she wrote to him from Moscow with cries for help ("for God's sake send money quickly"), and with instructions to "tear this letter up", lest Pavel find it.

By seventeen or eighteen, Anton was able to do some of what his father demanded, while making good use of his separation from family at the same time. His social life, flirtations and new experiences, flourished. He did well enough in school to graduate and to acquire his scholarship to University. He wrote a drama, *Fatherlessness*, alas long lost, and also a farce. In his letters he wrote believably of his loneliness for his parents and siblings. He did not founder, however, nor rebel and harden against them.

By late childhood, Anton had seemed able to withstand beatings, "tyrannies and lies," and keep his own counsel. He took advantage of whatever freedom and pleasures came his way. He earned some de facto respect from his father as a responsible helper. How did he do this? We can only say what did happen. Already in boyhood, Anton showed his creative and observant powers. He could entertain others—sometimes even his father—with bright, farcical portrayals of adults' hypocrisies, stupidities, self-delusions. There is surely great relief in such a gift, which offers both detachment and acceptable revenge. He had a companionship with his two older brothers that allowed them all new experiences away from home. They shared good health and strength as boys, for testing the world and making mischief. Later they remained honest friends—though not without storms and conflicts. They were never forced by home conditions into sabotage of each other.

At school, Anton found an atmosphere of respect. Corporal punishment was not allowed. These are only a few of the lifelines Anton found in childhood. Without enough of these, abused children cannot escape some of those psychic deformities, which Egor molded in Pavel. Pavel was full of anger, but not apparently aware of it. He could not show or receive affection. He seemed lacking in ordinary concern for his offspring. He was obsessive, argumentative, tyrannical. Pavel's range of experience was narrow, and his religious dictums "received from God" were often as harsh as his own father's orders. He was usually lonely. I think Anton was aware that this heritage threatened him, too.

Such fears he spoke of only rarely, and to intimates, in his letters. Thus, to Suvorin, and to his wife-to-be, Olga, he wrote that he was indeed a hot tempered man, trying hard to curb this. Usually he permitted no doubt, that he and his brothers could rid themselves of the aimlessness, and coarseness, that surrounded them in their early poverty. Yet there was an edge, sometimes, to his humor about this. Once, as he held the family cat, Fiodor Timofeich, which Aleksandr had rescued from a freezing latrine in Moscow, Anton remarked of the family, "Who would have thought that such genius would come out of an earth closet?" And there was no humor in the corrosive self-loathing Anton could express during periods of depression. At thirty-two, for example, he wrote to Suvorin, "I am apathetic and bored with myself . . . I ought to have a bath in sulfuric acid, flay off my skin, and then grow a new hide."[7]

It speaks for the sincerity of Chekhov's early determination to be "well bred" and compassionate, that his occasional lapses can startle us. Why are they so surprising? I believe they are unexpected sightings of how much deep anger he carried from boyhood. There is verbal violence, for example, in his descriptions to Suvorin of the St. Petersburg writers he loathed. He called the literati not people, but "some kind of walking mildew." "Ever since my conversation with that writer, I've had the sort of aftertaste in my mouth I'd get if, instead of vodka, I'd had a shot of ink mixed with flies."[8] He was able to conceal this hatred, however, in his actual behavior.

The "lapses" show us how grimly he'd set himself to avoid intrusion from other people. He would ignore others' needs, or even punish them, if he felt his personal freedom was in danger.

For example, Anton was a teaser. This was most often comical and affectionate. He gave his brothers, friends and lovers, caricaturing names. In his letters to women, he made melodramatic fun of their attachment to him. (The one exception to this is in his loving letters to Olga.) This could be cruelly hurtful. Lika Mizinova, who yearned desperately for Anton's love, was moved to write in one response, "What a savage you are, Anton..."[9]

He was elusive. A reader of Chekhov biographies finds it hard to follow some of his trips and travels—despite the guiding efforts of extensive research. Anton often made sudden changes in his plans, and notified nobody. Sometimes he was depressed, restless; or simply sick of the importunings of would-be companions. His family complained of his unannounced disappearances. They had then the full burden of the work at home, and he often left them without enough money. It is painful to read of Suvorin and the elderly Grigorovich, in 1889, waiting and watching for Anton for days, in Vienna, where he had promised to join them. He, meanwhile, had opted for a boat trip in the Crimea. Grigorovich never quite forgave Anton this. Grigorovich's complaint to Suvorin is interesting: "he hasn't been treating us like a European . . . He's a Slav, disorderly with no firm support to help him control himself . . . I'm now angry with him."[10]

Chekhov's indifference to his intimates' feelings was not the rule; but the exceptions were startling. Sometimes he used friends recognizably in his literary works. He himself shunned any public focus on his private life. Yet he seemed surprised, and unrepentant, at others' fury. There was an early instance of this indiscretion during Anton's medical school days. He and Kolya published a caricature sketch of his Taganrog relatives at a family wedding they'd attended. This disrupted family connections for years. Later, in his story "The Grasshopper," Chekhov included bits of many of his friends, and whole unflattering portrayals of others. (Revenge for recent wounds suffered in love was probably one motive.) Some broke off friendship with Anton forever, over this, and some for several years. The artist Levitan wanted to challenge him to a duel. Lika reproached Anton for hurting others. She acknowledged he did not actually intend this; but he didn't seem to care how other people were affected.

Even his sister Masha, his lifelong willing helpmate, allowed herself to remark to some of Anton's friends that "there is nothing more selfish than talent and genius."[11]

Anton's great effort at self-definition, at age sixteen to nineteen, was to my mind clear indication that he sensed inner threats to his integrity and his future. He took steps to plan for adulthood with balance.

This was an early age, in any time or culture, for a boy to spell out his spiritual life goals so farsightedly. This period of separation from his family, while still enjoying some adolescent freedom, mixed with loneliness, in his home town, must have provided just what he needed. He could take the measure of his past and imagine his future. In a later letter to Suvorin, he describes the vision: "the son of a serf, a former grocer, choir boy, schoolboy and university student, raised on respect for rank, kissing the priests' hands, worshipping the ideas of others, and giving thanks for every piece of bread, receiving frequent whippings, making the rounds as a tutor without galoshes, brawling, torturing animals, enjoying dinner at the houses of rich relatives, needlessly hypocritical before God and man merely to acknowledge his own insignificance —write about how this young man squeezes the slave out of himself drop by drop and how, on waking up one fine morning, he finds that the blood coursing through his veins is no longer the blood of a slave, but that of a real human being."[12]

The primary tenet of this task was to be his "personal freedom": "the most absolute freedom imaginable, freedom from violence and lies, no matter what form the latter two take." In the 1888 letter to the poet Aleksei Plescheev in which he states this, the full sentence begins, "My holy of holies is the human body, health, intelligence, talent, inspiration, love and the most absolute freedom imaginable... (etc.)"[13] This is a list of matters most dear to him, which he will honor and develop within the walled protection of his freedom. "Decency" is on this list too. As Charles Du Bos commented, "Decency ever so closely allies in the case of Chekhov to the notion of personal freedom."[14] Anton amply spelled out "decency" in an 1886 letter of scolding and instructions to Kolya. He says that well bred people respect other individuals; are therefore always indulgent, gentle, polite and compliant. "They do not throw a tantrum over a hammer or lost eraser." Their compassion "extends beyond beggars and cats. They are hurt even by things the naked eye can't see." They pay their debts. "They are candid and fear lies like the plague . . . they cultivate their aesthetic sensibilities ... they cannot stand [to] see a slit in the wall teeming with bedbugs . . . they require spontaneity, elegance, compassion . . ."[15] This description of good breeding reads, of course, like a thinly veiled exhortation to avoid the ways of their father. It also stands as a thoughtful vision of a good life, which Anton had set against his childhood experiences. And it is a picture of that person whom Chekhov became.

Chekhov's stated purposes rouse associations to religious life. Certainly, long after he lost belief in God, he always acknowledged his love of church words and ceremonies, and the tolling of bells. Not for nothing does he use the words "credo"; "my holy of holies"; "they are hurt even by things the naked eye can't see." For me, the life principles he stated and restated have an almost physical presence. As at the monastery of Akhtyrka, where Anton took solace with his family after Kolya's death, as at the Novodevichie monastery where Chekhov is buried, a high thick wall surrounds the life within. His soul's wall was his insistence on absolute personal freedom. Inside it he lived as richly as possible—creating classic literary works, performing charitable and healing acts as a physician, supporting his family, loving fine things, and friendships, and the company of women. The perimeter was strict, however. Women who might entrap him were excluded. His consumptive illness was denied as long as possible—like the Tatar at the gates. Its entry would bring dependency, not freedom.

Accounts have been left, of the bustle of life within the walls of actual monasteries in the past. Eating, drinking, studying, singing, loving, flourished there as anywhere else. Flexible but firm principles of the Order, however, kept the communal life in balance. I think Anton's inner life was like this. His outward life too partook of the monastic. He early became secular abbot of the family, as well as son and brother. As such, he oversaw a home for the family and for sojourning friends. Comfort, routine, gardens, and a good many pleasures, were there for all. From this enclave, Anton Pavlovich often strayed but always returned. He lived with his parents in a manner dictated by his principles. (To Suvorin he joked, "he has a noble family that needs his protection".[16]) He was affectionate towards his overanxious mother, and hid all worrisome matters from her. He was civil to his father, despite the many things Pavel did and said which continued to cause domestic troubles. His sister Masha ran the household according to his wishes. He praised her, and brought her gifts, and effectively discouraged her marrying and leaving. Anton was the young patriarch at home; keeping a modest demeanor. He taught precepts for living to his younger siblings; techniques for sensible buying, and avoidance of debt, to his mother and sister. Many visiting friends praised the warmth of Anton's home. We do notice the sexual taboos within the sanctuary, however. His sister was not his wife: he did not share with her his doubts or dreams or passions. And he did not seem to wish to leave this home, as real-life husband or father—until, so late, and ill, he met Olga Knipper.

A second key protector of balance appeared in young Chekhov's choosing of a dual career: literature, and medicine. This seemed to begin without planning or fanfare. He kept both professions, however, for most of his life. Let us look first at the history of Anton's tilts to one side or the other, as the inner gyroscope dictated, as he went along.

Doctoring was his "wife," he said, and writing his "mistress." If the one disappointed or bored him, he would find more pleasure with the other. He said, "This is irregular but at least not monotonous and neither suffers from my infidelity."[17] These words reflect the adaptiveness of Anton's arrangements with himself. He could be aware of his needs for change or escape, without suffering heavy guilt.

In medical school, his learning to be a doctor was paramount. He wrote comic stories chiefly as a source of income—a paltry one at first, then gradually more lucrative. He described those stories as "comic piffle"—perhaps true, often, because Chekhov was twenty and the stories relied on "secondhand traditions and second-rate devices." By age twenty-five, he wrote deeper and better constructed stories. In 1884, as Chekhov graduated as a full-fledged general practitioner, we note that the "mistress" was also taken seriously. Anton saw to it that his *Tales of Melpomene* was published just then for the reading public.

He started practice that summer in Dr. Arkhangelsky's Chikino Hospital; meanwhile writing "The Huntsman," a fine, Turgenev-like story. In the fall, he opened practice from his home in Moscow. He held office hours four days a week, and also attended to the medical care of prostitutes, and did autopsies, to earn more money. In quiet office hours, and at his country home in Babkino, he wrote such works as "On the Harm of Tobacco"; "Grief"; "Artistry."

By age twenty-six, Anton's literary work began to be recognized. Suvorin, an influential publisher, accepted his stories and befriended him. The revered writer Grigorovich also expressed his admiration. Anton then vowed to take his gift seriously. The literary world opened to him: there were trips to Moscow, and invitations for new friends to his Babkino home. Despite this busy social life—with little time even to sleep—Anton continued to dispense medicines, and to write new stories for *Fragments*. From Babkino, Anton wrote, "I'm seeing a lot of patients, children with rickets and old folks with rashes. There's one old lady with erisypelas on her arm."[18] The next summer, the family began to rent an estate in Sumy in the Ukraine. There, Anton helped the timorous doctor Elena Lintvariova with her diagnoses and surgical procedures.

He continued to diagnose and treat many of his literary friends: Grigorovich, Suvorin, Leikin, etc., as well as family members. He helped Dr. Arkhangelsky with his study of Russia's psychiatric institutions. He also wrote several stories, and completed his play, *Ivanov*. Neither mistress nor wife was abandoned. Chekhov wrote to Suvorin, "I feel more alert and more satisfied with myself when I think of myself as having two occupations instead of one."[19] Literature was his major source of income: he was now well paid by his editors. So for economic reasons as well as inspiration, he wrote prolifically. He created "The Steppe," a masterpiece, during this time.

Loneliness, however, and revulsion for the literary world, were welling up in Anton. Alongside his own inner pressures, the increasing sickness and dissipation of his comrade Levitan and his brother Kolya may have darkened his mood. Aleksandr's wife, Anna, too, was dying of tuberculosis. Aleksandr had a sudden hysterical blindness. All four beseeched Anton for help. At twenty-seven, he wrote a suicidal letter to Aleksandr about his own "moral vomiting." Yet he continued his many activities. Even the initial hostile reaction in Moscow to the opening of *Ivanov* did not unbalance him for long. *Ivanov*, indeed, is a vivid example of Chekhov's ability to rely on both medicine and literature. He is objective and psychologically correct, in his presentation of Ivanov's slide into depression. And his artistry is not skewed by emotional difficulties of his own. The critic Charles Du Bos has best summed up this artistic achievement: ". . . it is not Chekhov himself who is depressed—or at least if he has in him a potential vein of depression, his fine and clear balance outweighs it—it is his characters who are depressed, which is a different matter; and this would more readily explain how his works can have a bracing effect (if not because of the characters' vitality, at least because of the will to vitality in the author who stands behind them)."[20]

Kolya's death in June of 1889 did truly dim Anton Pavlovich's sense of well-being. He had lost an early, gifted, ally. He could not save Kolya from tuberculosis by medical ministrations—and in fact had left him to Aleksandr's nursing care in the final days, defecting from his hopeless doctoring on an ill-timed excursion. He alone of the family could not cry at Kolya's funeral. And Kolya had died of the disease already well entrenched in Anton himself.

For awhile, Anton spent time in Moscow with a series of adoring actresses. His play, *The Wood Demon*, failed. (Later, he could use and improve much of its material in *Uncle Vanya.*) He wrote "A Dreary Story": again able to transform his own sense of alienation into great literature. But he was truly drawing away from his "mistress" now. He'd come to feel that the St. Petersburg literary giants "serve evil", were "jaded, apathetic, idly philosophizing,"[21] and shunned their company. He could not find new stories in himself; took to passing the time on editing tasks Suvorin gave him. It was medical science to which he turned for hope, at last. He decided to journey as a physician to the penal Island of Sakhalin. As he prepared, his depression lifted.

His project—to take a census of all persons and their circumstances in the remote Siberian penal colony, and to write an objective account of it for the edification of the Russian people—was a steep tilt indeed away from literature. It was his writing fame which made the trip politically possible, of course; and hosts along the way were eager for contact with the famous author. Chekhov hewed to his medical role, however—diagnosing, lancing abscesses, posing the medical questions, everywhere on the island. And not long after his return home, he moved the family to a new country estate, Melikhovo, where he set up medical practice at once. What he did there as Dr. Chekhov has been described in the previous chapter. He also wrote voluminously and well during the Melikhovo years. The gyroscope had returned, it seems, to its active upright balance. It was perhaps overactive. Even on the train returning to Melikhovo, after the humiliating failure of the premier of *The Seagull* in St. Petersburg, he spent the hours of travel planning for committee meetings on roads and school buildings, treatment of sick peasants, and brooding over the major story, "Peasants," which had begun to take shape.

Six months later, acute illness felled Anton. With definitive hospital diagnosis of his consumption, and with as much medical supervision from then on as Chekhov would allow, he was forced to give up his medical practice. He still related to many old and new friends as a physician, treating and advising them. In Nice, where he went for his own health, Chekhov soon allowed his fellow boarders at the Pension Russe to use him as doctor. His financial and organizational help to social causes continued. And in his letter of 1899 to Dr. Rossolimo is a powerful statement of his allegiance in all things to the "scientific method." We know, however, that his great work in these last years was done in literature. It included "The Lady with the Little Dog," "The Bishop"; *Three Sisters*, and *The Cherry Orchard*.

An important major shift occurred for Chekhov, finally, in the last three years of his life. He married Olga Knipper. He had at last been able to fall in love, and remain so. He spoke of his wish for a child, for the first time. Though the couple had months-long separations, and left much unshared or hidden between them, it is plain in his letters that Anton could reveal many pains, and desires, to this woman. He looked to Olga for happiness and comfort—no longer to his family of origin, where intimacy was so limited. This long-resisted shift in balance helped center him, to the end; as his dual careers faded.

As a boy, Anton faced the classic challenges of any child growing up. He must tame his aggression, and discourage his dependency. He must learn to keep self respect and also respect others. He is a sexual being. And so on. We have some sense already of what poor soil his parents could provide for some of this growth. Yet Anton developed quite well, with grace and balance. He did not hide away and wither, like his own "Man in the Case." He was not as prone to drunkenness, outburst and debauchery as his older brothers who were also abused. (He had a major artistic talent; but both of them were very gifted as well.) We cannot answer most of our questions about what formed him: the vectors in his childhood family are untraceable, except in the crudest way. In retrospect, it can at least be seen that he met many of his own needs for growth by the choices—and luck—he found in his two professions.

Being a doctor earned Chekhov some degree of social status beyond his forebears. It earned him some, but not much, money; but that was really of his own choosing. He wanted an independent consulting room, and one he could shut down without interference when he so decided. He wanted to treat poor people. All this could be managed because he earned by writing. It was a complicated matter, this earning a living, for this complicated man. Anton kept himself and his family reasonably housed and fed—but often went into debt over traveling, or buying goods and estates, or building schools, beyond the money in his account. Since his literary works were highly valued, he could then work hard to turn out stories, or could ask Suvorin for an advance. Perhaps Anton had inherited Pavel's love of gourmet fare and generous hospitality in his "bourgeois drawing room," in the prosperous days in the grocery store. Unlike his father, however, Anton always repaid his debts. As he wrote to his brother at twenty-six, well-bred men must "respect the property of others and therefore pay their debts."[22] Anton worried considerably about all this. He told Suvorin that when he asked for an advance, he then suffered "fear that people as decent as myself might get the idea that I'm publishing so often only for the sake of lucre."[23] He wrote, "I don't love money enough for medicine..."[24] His own standard seemed to require that he practice medicine gratis. He rejoiced, during the cholera epidemic, that he worked tirelessly for the zemstvo, but did not accept payment, nor spend even a kopeck of zemstvo money. Sometimes he regretted this a little. "Yesterday I treated a boy and declined the six rubles his mommy tried to slip me. Now I'm sorry I declined."[25]

If our balance in life is less a matter of solid engineering than of continual dynamic rearrangements, then Chekhov's ways with money are a fine example. Basically, his "mistress," literature, provided for him generously in the style he loved. He could be selfless with his "wife." His wealthy friend Suvorin gave reliable, fatherly financial backup when there was need. So Anton had created a flexible way of living that furnished him with what his childhood had not. His letters show that he was not always pleased with his own lapses. By the end of his life, however, he was fully adult and parental, in his careful financial provision for mother, sister and wife.

The science and objectivity of medicine was dear to Chekhov in many ways. This mode of thought was only then coming into its own in Russia. It promised new solutions for the nation's poverty, disease and ignorance. For Anton personally, it was a counterforce to Pavel's blind religious fervor, and to the superstition of his peasant forebears. Humanistic medical practice, with strict attention to what is actually possible, and what the goals and methods of intervention should be, was the right "temperature" for Chekhov. He usually avoided public activism to right social wrongs. He shunned most displays of zeal, or faith, in fact—be they in love affairs or in religious observance. Daily work as a doctor did sometimes bring him joy. Telling Suvorin about fighting an epidemic, he wrote: "I was both horrified and delighted . . . In the good old days when people fell ill and died by the thousands, no one would even have dreamed of the astounding victories taking place before our very eyes."[26] More prosaically, Anton sometimes treated friends to a glimpse of his pleasures in practice. "I have just poured castor oil from little bottles into a large one. A pleasant occupation."[27] (To Suvorin, just after completing *The Sea Gull*). To his brother he wrote from Melikhovo with happy practicality: "Keep well and bring some corks, the ordinary bottle ones, and some pharmacists ones but not too many."[28] He included two drawings of corks.

Chekhov could make distance from friends as he felt it necessary, by emphasizing his medical credentials. He told Suvorin about the medical fight against cholera; then added, "It's a shame you're not a doctor and can't share my pleasure, that is, deeply sense and understand and appreciate everything that is happening."[29] In his frequent doctoring of literary friends and amorous women, he sometimes teased these patients about their symptoms. He was not above telling one friend about another's medical weaknesses, as literary gossip. The patient might show an overconcern about health, or be afraid to take the arsenic pills Chekhov had prescribed. Some of his superior attitude was possibly in reaction to denigration of doctors by some of his friends. His poet friend Palmin, for example, who asked Chekhov to treat him, and seldom paid, through the years, called Anton "Mr. Rest-in-Peace"; address, "Dead Lane, Coffin House, Cross-Kisser's flat, which is for any doctor, especially a young doctor, a suitable address."[30]

Medical practice was notably useful, like his literary work, in enabling Anton to be well-bred while never losing contact with his grimy peasant roots. His lancing of abscesses, treatment of broken limbs and heads and far-gone cancerous growths—all those night calls to visit the sick and dying in their smoky village huts—kept him observant and truthful about the poor. In many of his letters, and of course shining through his stories, there is pride in his understanding. Anton enjoyed doing autopsies. He performed one at age twenty-four, in a village, with anxious peasants surrounding him and the dead drunken man. He described the ignorance and superstitions of these watchers with relish, in a letter to a friend. Meanwhile, he knew he was performing a socially useful function there, all the same.

In his childhood and youth, Anton Pavlovich lived amongst all kinds of dirt. This was literal, in the cockroach-infested back rooms of the grocery store; and metaphorical, as in "dirty dealing," foul language, and the soiling of virtue and reputation going on in his family and the surround. In his youthful credo, Anton vowed to cultivate his aesthetic sensibilities. It is not surprising that as a doctor, he rejoiced in the "cleanup" of disease that disinfection made possible. He never removed himself, however, from dealings with peasants, or women in brothels who "smell of horse sweat." He gladly led the local fight against cholera, with its stink and misery. That is why we readers have "Peasants," and "Sorrow." His realism kept Chekhov himself in balance. He wanted to remain "ordinary," as he told Suvorin—not to be a literary celebrity.

Women puzzled Chekhov; or frightened him. He wanted to define their "exact nature." Are they less creative and intelligent than men, and if so why?

In medical school, freshly imbued with "objectivity," he hoped for awhile to collaborate with Aleksandr on a scientific study. This, *A History of Sexual Authority*, would follow Darwin's lead. They would trace the natural history of living species, to determine if the male's dominance is inevitable. Anton guessed it was not: if the female is liberated from a life of caring for the young, she may grow to be equal. He did believe that men are *presently* superior to women. "[She is] passive . . . never and nowhere is she superior to man in the political and sociological sense . . . she is a good doctor but in the sphere of *creative activity* she is a goose . . . the perfect organism *creates*, and woman, as yet, has not created anything."[31]

Five years later, as a young doctor, Anton described to Suvorin how he helped Dr. Elena Lintvariova in her medical practice at Sumy. He said he was much braver than she in prescribing healthy doses of medicine, and in looking calmly at poor prognoses. This woman physician was "infinitely kind and loving," but overanxious, and "where death is obvious and inevitable, my doctor friend reacts quite unprofessionally."[32] Anton's history with his own overwhelmed mother must surely come to mind.

It can be noted that Chekhov judged women writers' works by these same standards. Those who asked for his mentorship were sternly warned against sentimentality and vagueness. He gave his highest praise to his friend, Maria Kiseliova, for a story of hers: ". . . there are roughnesses, but the conciseness and masculine manner of the story redeem everything."[33]

Whatever his reasons, Chekhov's letters give many examples of his pleasure at being decisive and "hard hearted" when that is needed. He enjoyed the manliness of his emergency zemstvo work. He treated the genitourinary diseases of prostitutes calmly. He challenged the tsar's government by visiting its penal colony and telling about it.

There is some evidence of a hesitant, shy side of Chekhov, which he tried to erase or hide. His classmate and friend, Grigori Rossolimo, described him in medical school as exceptionally shy. His mentor in early hospital practice, Dr. Arkhangelsky, said, "sometimes a kind of hesitancy appeared in his manner."[34] Not long afterwards, in his new Moscow practice, he was so upset by the death of a woman patient from typhoid that he briefly considered giving up doctoring. Such moments and qualities are common in doctors' lives. Most learn from their medical experience to become more confident—as Dr. Chekhov did. I mention them only as points along the way, as he looked for his own balance of forthrightness and reserve, of masculine and feminine. Manliness without bullying, softness with staying power, were in his credo.

Lastly, I will mention the love and admiration given to Dr. Chekhov by patients. He does not discuss this in his letters, except to complain of it as a doctor's burden. But evidence suggests that Anton became a "legend" in the area of his practice in Melikhovo. A pleased patient wrote in a letter, "We have a doctor near here the like of whom you won't find in Moscow . . . he is well loved by everyone. He doesn't even charge me for my medicine."[35] A man reported, ". . . my wife when she was old kept going to him for treatment. He cured her. Then I fell ill and he attended to me. I gave him money but he wouldn't take it. So I say, 'Anton Pavlovich, my dear chap, what are you doing?—you're not stupid and you know your business' but he just kept on laughing."[36]

Such tributes are payment to doctors for their labors and inconveniences. The love has been earned. It has no complicated strings. It also comes from those who have experienced the quality of the doctor personally and truthfully. All of the above would be pleasing to Anton Chekhov. It stands in contrast to much of the adulation he received because his literary works were famous. He was uneasy, or furious, when admirers spotted him. He sensed envy hidden in the admiration of his literary peers, except for intimate friends. Praise from his medical colleagues, as from his patients, was a different matter, down-to-earth and well earned. The zemstvo, for example, made a formal proposition "thanking Dr. A P Chekhov for his unselfish and useful part in the struggle against the threatening cholera epidemic in the Serpukhov District." Correspondence with his old friend Rossolimo has a friendly, collegial intimacy, which centers on medical matters and their common past. Chekhov wrote to him more forthrightly than to his editors and fellow artists, with of course exceptions. One can understand the ballast his career as doctor gave Chekhov, for his literary voyage.

It is both odd and true, that I cannot assess the contributions of Anton Chekhov's writing career to his satisfaction and balance. Odd, because his literary gift is what prompts the wish to know him. True, because I can find no letter or memoir of him that helps. He described to good friends some times of doubt and difficulty in his writing. The rest—his daily and lifelong experience of sitting alone with paper and pen—lies unknown. I will add only these few thoughts.

In his medical work, Chekhov could question and test some of his suppositions about women that were so often on his mind. In his many life experiences with women, he roved and learned. And in his stories and plays? Here are the wonderful fruits of his observations. Some of the female portraits he drew we recognize in accounts of Anton's personal life. He knew well several sets of "three sisters," for example—each with a body, a temperament, talents and wishes, that led her to a separate fate within a family way of living. Most of the fictional women we haven't met before. We know at once about all of them, that they are exceptionally truly drawn. There is Olga Semionovna, "The Darling," with her "plump, fine shoulders"; Anna Sergeevna, "The Lady with the Little Dog," described by such different detail. The young Anton, who imitated characters so ably in home dramatics, perfected this gift in the written word. He remained in the business of entertainment. But now the standard of truthfulness was very high.

The interweaving of Chekhov's scientific self with his literary identity was a great source of strength. He told Dr. Rossolimo that his study of medicine "significantly broadened the scope of my observations", and that when he had no firm data, "I have preferred not writing at all."[37] The beauty of Chekhov's work rests upon this, I believe. What he left out, having "no data," hangs in the air around. We are allowed to join him in his scrupulousness, and find we do not need to ask for more.

Chekhov wrote "The Student" at age thirty-four. This story is short and spare. It describes a young student priest walking home for Easter, through a still-wintry countryside. He meets two country women by their fire. He tells them the story of Peter's denying Jesus thrice, then weeping—on just such a freezing night, by a fire. Only homely details of weather and terrain, of the women's responses and of the student's thoughts, are given. But somehow, through the peasant women and the immature young man, we readers are included in a religious experience. And we know Chekhov, the "irreligious man," joins us.

For me, this is his most poetic story. Let me end our subject of Chekhov's balance with it. Here, Anton Pavlovich was able to create a simple, self-contained happening as a poem does. Around this, the imagination of the reader comes eagerly to life, and provides the many meanings of the tale. The student of the story has done just this, too, without conscious intention; standing by the fire with the listening women. Chekhov has drawn the student, the peasant women, ourselves and himself, into a perfectly centered space.

I know nothing about Chekhov's conscious desire to communicate through his art; nor with whom he most wanted this sharing. He did not discuss it. Still, we can boldly suppose that like other poets, he needed these encounters between writer and reader that enlarge and center them both.

V.
The White Plague

The thread of tubercular illness is woven into Chekhov's life from its beginning. He might slightly rearrange its pattern—ignore it, aggravate it by hard living, or soothe it by rest—but the disease was a force beyond Anton's balancing maneuvers. It belonged to the Angel of Death. For Anton Pavlovich, in his historical period, it was even more inescapable than the oppression of the Tsarist regime. The "personal freedom" he always insisted upon was gradually taken away by this impersonal force; though he resisted, and adjusted, to the end.

Almost nothing has changed from Chekhov's time to ours, in the clinical presentation of active tuberculosis. What I write here is true for him and for ourselves. For that matter, nothing has changed from the times of Hippocrates and Galen. Chekhov read their superb clinical descriptions in medical school.

The disease gains entry to the human lungs when droplets of sputum from nearby infected persons are inhaled. An infant or child who breathes in the tubercle bacilli this way may have no observable symptoms. Perhaps there is a short period of fever, which passes. Sometimes it happens that he or she may die then, of massive infection or poor resistance. Anton's niece Mosia, and his baby sister Evgenia, may have died this way. Adolescents and early adults have traditionally made up the majority of patients. Only recently, since medications are available to lower the overall risk to the young, older people make up a higher percentage. In chronic pulmonary tuberculosis like Chekhov's, the bacilli live and multiply in "tubercles," protective casings they create within the lungs. They may destroy small blood vessels there, causing bleeding into the bronchi, and the bloody sputum so frequently observed. They may spread, by invading the blood stream, to other organs. Bones and joints, brain, skin, intestines and other body parts can be affected. Classically, the person with chronic disease has bouts of hectic fever, progressive emaciation, night sweats, cough, spitting of blood. There are better, and worse, periods through weeks and months. The probable occurrence of early death, often after some years, is the result of invasion and destruction of the organs, overburdening of the heart, and general exhaustion of physical resources.

Much of this was illustrated in Anton Chekhov's own words, through the years, written in letters to friends or in his notebooks, about his own condition. A few comments of friends about him are included here too—his observers' view.

Age twenty-eight, to Plescheev. "I am depressed. I have a hemorrhage. It is probably nothing, but still it is unpleasant."[1]

Same year, to Suvorin. "But all this frightens me only when there is hemorrhage: in blood coming from the mouth there is something ominous, as in the flare of a fire." [2]

Age twenty-nine, to Plescheev. "My holy of holies is the human body, health, intelligence, talent, inspiration, love, and the most absolute freedom."[3]

Age thirty, to Suvorin, on beginning the journey to Sakhalin. "Only the lack of sleep, the jolting and the fasting, brought on spitting of blood when I coughed, and this depressed my spirits."[4]

Same year, to Suvorin, on return from that journey. "I now have a happy feeling as though I had not been away from home at all. I am well and thriving to the marrow of my bones."[5]

Age thirty-one, to Suvorin, on the death of a mutual friend. "Death is slowly gathering her own. She knows her business."[6]

Same year, to Suvorin. "I continue to grow stupid, dull, indifferent, withering and coughing, and I already begin to think that my health will not recover. But all that is in the hands of God. Remedies and anxieties about my physical existence arouse in me a feeling akin to disgust. I will not be doctored. I shall take the waters and quinine, but I am not going to be sounded . . ."[7]

Four days later, to Suvorin. "My health is improving. My cough is less, I feel stronger, my mood is livelier, and there is sunrise in my head. I wake up in the morning in a happy spirit, go to bed with no gloomy thoughts, and at dinner I am not peevish and do not say rude things to mother."[8]

A few weeks later, to Shmagin. "It seems to me that I am dried and warped like an old cupboard, and that if I go on living in Moscow next season, and give myself up to scribbling excesses, Galgarovsky will read an excellent poem to welcome my entrance into that country place where there is neither sitting nor standing nor sneezing but only lying down and nothing more!"[9]

Age thirty-three, to Suvorin. Chekhov had not yet publicly admitted to having consumption. "Last night I had severe palpitation of the heart, but I was not alarmed, although it was hard to breathe, and I took up *Pascal* [Zola's novel]... the novel is very good. And so, I repeat, I was not frightened by the palpitation, because all such sensations as shocks, lapses, sinkage of the heart and the like are extremely deluding. The enemy who kills the body comes usually imperceptibly, wearing a mask, as when, for instance, you are ill with consumption and it seems to you that it is not consumption, but a trifle merely . . . It follows that that is terrible of which you are not afraid; but that which arouses your apprehensions is not terrible . . . All-healing nature, in killing us, at the same time artfully deceives us, as a nurse does a child when she carries it away from the drawing room to bed . . ."[10]

Age thirty-four, to Aleksandr. “I do not want to write, and indeed it’s hard to combine a desire to live and a desire to write.”[11]

At age thirty-seven, Anton was seriously ill, and hospitalized. That year, several friends described him to others.

“His face was yellow and he looked worn out. He coughed frequently and wrapped himself in his blanket as if cold although the wind was inexplicably warm.”[12] (Shcheglov).

“I think he has no idea of the danger of his state, although to my mind he is a typical consumptive.” (Kovalevsky)[13]

“[On his travels he liked] churchyards and circuses with clowns.”[14] (Suvorin).

Age thirty-eight, to Lidia Avilova. “[The writing process is now like] eating cabbage soup from which a cockroach has just been removed.”[15] At that time, however, Chekhov wrote “Gooseberries,” “The Man in the Case,” and other great stories.

Age thirty-nine, to Dr. Rossolimo. “I’m in Yalta, in exile, a beautiful exile, perhaps, but exile just the same. Life goes by drearily...” [16]

Age forty, to Batiushkov. “I am dull here. I am sick of it, and I have a feeling as though I have been thrown overboard. And the weather’s bad too, and I am not well . . .”[17]

Same year, to Lidia Avilova. “I am nearly well; I am ill from time to time, but not often and only because I am old—the bacilli have nothing to do with it. And when I see a lovely woman now I smile in an aged way, and drop my lower lip—that’s all.”[18]

Age forty-two, to Balmont. “It is wonderful in Yalta, perfectly summer weather—and that is bad: all night long the cats are yelling, the dogs are howling, and one dreams of burial vaults; during the day the sun shines brightly and memories haunt one, and one longs for the cold and the people of the North.”[19]

Age forty-three, to his wife Olga. "I sit unwashed like a *samoyed* [savage]. I even begin to growl. You ask me if I at least wash my neck. Yes, I wash my neck but the rest of me is as dirty as an old galosh."[20]

Chekhov had once written in his notebook that "one should be mentally clear, morally pure, and physically tidy."

That same year, Bunin described a visit to Chekhov in his Yalta family. "'You are not feeling well, Antosha?', his mother or sister would say, seeing him sitting all day with his eyes shut. 'I?', he would answer quietly—'oh, it's nothing. I have a little headache.'"[21]

Age forty-four, to Lidia Avilova. "Above all, be cheerful; don't look at life so much as a problem—it is, most likely, far simpler. And whether it—life, of which we know nothing—is worth all the agonizing reflections which wear out our Russian wits, is a question."[22]

In June, that year, to Masha from Badenweiler. "And so tell Mother and everyone who is interested that I am getting better, or indeed have already gotten better."[23]

Also in June, to Masha. "I long to go from here to Lake Como and stay there a short time. The Italian lakes are famous for their beauty..."[24]

Also in June, to Masha. "Evidently my digestion is hopelessly ruined. It is scarcely possible to cure it by anything but fasting—that is, eating nothing—and that's the end of it. And the only remedy for the asthma is not moving."[25]

Anton Pavlovich died on July 2nd.

The "white plague," tuberculosis, has ebbed and crested in human society since ancient times, and appeared almost everywhere in the world. Under conditions of human poverty, crowding, industrialization, social upheaval, it becomes epidemic. In better times it is endemic: cases are fewer, and strike those most vulnerable. In the 1950's, at last, medication was developed which could arrest tuberculosis. In 1900, in the

United States, it took second place in the nation's causes of death; while in 2002, its mortality rate was at all time low of 5.2 cases / 100,000 people. Its causative bacillus, mycobacterium tuberculosis var. hominis, however, has recently shown world-wide ability to develop resistance to drugs. Revised medications have been needed—and also massive public health efforts to see that patients receive enough medicine, and for long enough, to arrest the disease and prevent spread to others. Today this is seldom possible in poor or war-torn areas of the world. So tuberculosis renews its ravages.

Chekhov had his own reasons, as a young doctor, to deny that consumption was the probable cause of his recurrent cough bleeding from the lungs. No effective treatment for tuberculosis had yet been found. Even the wisest specialists could do no more than prescribe changes of climate, or diet; this usually availed little, as Anton Pavlovich knew. And consider the weight of his family history. His own mother's symptoms of probable tuberculosis were described in a letter of Pavel's, a year before Anton's birth. His uncle Vanya, aunt Fenichka, cousin Elizaveta, brother Kolya, sister-in-law Anna, and probably his niece Mosia, all died of it. Denial was at least an alternative to despair, for a man who insisted on living out a productive life without invalidism, as long as he could.

When Chekhov was a student and a young doctor, the x-ray had not yet been invented. Without that truth-teller to contradict him, Anton Pavlovich could speak off-handedly of his cough, the blood in his sputum, as "influenza," a touch of typhoid, or gastritis. He avoided any physician's examination that might disclose consolidation of disease in parts of his lungs. When Anton Pavlovich was in medical school, Dr. Robert Koch, in Germany, discovered that "mycobacterium tuberculosis var. hominis" is the cause of tuberculosis. Diagnosis could be definitive, when these bacilli were found in a patient's sputum. Some older Russian doctors did not really believe this. The scientific young Dr. Chekhov, however, did. It was a truth that finally trapped him in his own diagnosis in 1897, when he was hospitalized. In a light-toned letter to his friend Schechtel even a little earlier, he did not deny it: ". . . but sorry I can't marry just now, because, firstly, I have the bacilli in me, very dubious tenants."[26] This was a rare admission; made perhaps only to silence his friend's urging that he marry.

Probably, before roentgenograms, there was incomplete understanding of consumption's usual course. The first encounter with the bacilli is in infancy or childhood, in most cases. Germs breathed in which enter the child's lungs, also enter some of the body's lymph nodes that protect against disease. Most children show few symptoms at this time. Later, only small calcified lymph nodes in which the bacilli were trapped are seen on x-ray, marking the past infection. (This is known as the "primary complex.") Adults who fall ill of consumption are usually being reinfected from these dormant, walled-off germs in their own lungs—now reactivated in a time of bodily stress. If Chekhov and his colleagues did not know this clearly, it may account for his seeming omission of the family's babies from his conscientious doctoring of his relatives. For example, he scolded Aleksandr vigorously—with the authority his medical degree bestowed—about his chaotic and unsanitary family life. In these letters, however, there is no mention of the need to protect Aleksandr's baby, Mosia, from the germs of her actively tubercular mother, Anna. Mosia died before her first birthday, after a sickly period ending in coma, half-paralyzed. The baby's likeliest diagnosis is tuberculosis, invading the meninges or brain. Baby Anton, too, probably inhaled the bacilli exhaled by his tuberculous mother. But he was granted a longer life than Mosia.

Much as Anton coughed, for years, there is no mention of his isolating himself in periods of illness to protect family, friends or lovers. (He did cough into a handkerchief discreetly, and spit into a tidy bottle the discharge of blood and sputum.) He welcomed many consumptive friends to the family dinner table. The ubiquitousness of the disease must have discouraged any greater care. It is plain that Anton grieved long and hard over his brother Kolya's death by consumption. Yet he described Kolya's death, and Aleksandr's Anna's, as "not an event in human life," but "an ordinary thing."

Explanations and myths abounded for centuries before scientific evidence, about the reasons one person contracted this disease and others were spared. Theories varied by region, culture and historical time.

In New England in the year 1850, tuberculosis caused a quarter of all deaths—among rich and poor, gifted and ordinary, alike. Ideas about this disease were permeated for many literate citizens by "perverted sentimentalism," according to the historians, Renee and Jean Du Bos. They describe the "artificialities of the Romantic Era," so much cultivated to soften the harsh realities of life. With a paucity of down-to-earth knowledge, a tubercular young woman actually could become "a standard of feminine beauty."[27] Ellen Emerson, a Concord poet of the 1820's and first wife of Ralph Waldo Emerson, was seen by her readers in this way. Both she and her husband came from families decimated by tuberculosis; like Chekhov's. Her letters and poems, and Emerson's writings about her, make it clear that she was an intelligent, observant, courageous young woman, who only wished to be robustly healthy, not delicate. To be sure, her battle against consumption (she died at twenty) was a major subject of her writing. She wanted above all to "die well." Many readers who learned of her illness saw only the beauty—not the struggle and ugliness—in her short life. As Susan Sontag puts it, tuberculosis had become a "glamorous disease."[28] "Health might seem banal; even vulgar." The consumptive is seen as genteel, delicate, aristocratic, vulnerable, melancholic, interesting, and fashionable. Sontag wonders "how the reality of such a dreadful disease could be transformed so preposterously."[29]

It is notable that like Ellen Emerson herself, Chekhov never romanticized his own disease. Nor was it romanticized in his country generally. He did not consider himself, nor his tubercular friends and family members, to be glamorous or interesting in their illness. In Russia, tuberculosis was only a scourge: ugly, frightening, and as Chekhov said, "ordinary."

Chekhov sometimes used his intimate knowledge of consumption tellingly, in his stories. He did not, however, have a "tubercular muse" like Ellen's—in the sense of making the fate of his illness, with all its attendant imagery, a centrally recurring theme.

I speculate whether he bore resemblance to the tubercular Franz Kafka—different as they were in the tenor of their lives and in their literary approach. Kafka observed, "Illness is speaking for me because I have asked it to do so."[30] I understand this to mean that the painful impasses of his early life continued with him, and proved unresolvable and unspeakable. The misery and damage he had suffered could best be enacted, and witnessed by others, in the bodily agony of his tuberculosis. Anton's brother Kolya may have had such a view of his own physical destruction—though less consciously than Kafka's. Anton Pavlovich was unlike them. He suffered his sickness very privately, and seldom asked for help or witness. Still it strikes me that Kolya and Anton both reenacted, in their carelessness for their bodies, the harsh disregard they had suffered in childhood, and the chronic lack of timely care.

Those of us who grew up "literary" in the years before World War II, and read romantic accounts of the tuberculous

Milton, Keats, Robert Louis Stevenson, Katherine Mansfield, and Chopin, might be tempted to add Chekhov to the list. We half-believed that the genius of these artists was due to the specific and magic effect of the toxin of the tubercle bacillus. "Spes phthisica" was the medical name for what was considered a nearly universal happening in chronic tuberculosis. There would be periods of rapid inroads by disease, with depression and lassitude—then an alternate state of constant agitation, even frenzy—which in talented people might accelerate cognitive and aesthetic effort. If we still believed that consumption fostered the works of genius, however, Dr. E.D.Wittkower, Assoc. Professor of Psychiatry at McGill University, helped to dispel this idea as early as 1956. He undertook scientific investigation of this and other myths. He concluded, simply that "tuberculosis is a common disease, and therefore also occurs in men and women of genius."[31] The disease does not stimulate intellectual activities, but has actually a dulling effect on a person's intellect during the active stages. To be sure, "during the long and weary months of slow progress, tuberculosis for a variety of reasons may favor fantasy production and therefore, production in the field of poetry and painting."[32] Also, "the dreaded limitation of their span of life stimulates their productivity. 'I try to cram into a short span of life what it would take others a lifetime to do,' a patient said."[33] Anton Pavlovich did speak of this urgency, in letters. More often he complained bitterly of the dulling effect of his illness.

Are sufferers from tuberculosis more intelligent than the general population? Dr. Wittkower investigated that belief too. Testing several hundred patients in a municipal sanatorium, he concluded that there was no link between IQ and this disease. Only, because they were deprived by sickness of so many physical activities, patients were "apt to develop intellectual interests and activities not infrequently above the accepted standard of their social class."[34] Perhaps young Ellen Emerson used her poetic gift even more intensely, in her enforced physical inactivity. As to Chekhov, I find no evidence of this. His tactic was always to give himself as little chance to be inactive in illness as possible. He never mentioned any positive creative benefit in it. Healthy idleness, yes—and idling in beautiful, natural surroundings—were his stated personal necessities for "happiness." But happiness is another matter.

A third myth which Dr. Wittkower discusses is a perceived link between tuberculosis and mental illness. He found, indeed, a higher rate of tuberculosis in the mental hospitals of the 1950's than in the population at large. Hospitalized schizophrenic patients had the highest rate. He concluded, however, that the link here was not etiological, but was the result of the hospitalization. "Tuberculous psychotics seem to be a potent source of mass infection"[35]—careless of their coughs and spitting, and infecting many others in the close hospital air. Moreover, careful psychological studies of hundreds of patients led him to believe that "*no* specific personality type prevails in tuberculous patients."[36]

Many medical observers of the past left accounts of consumptives who alternated periods of rapid worsening of their chest symptoms, with amelioration of these but appearance of florid psychotic symptoms. Benjamin Rush, our valued eighteenth century American physician, wrote: "It is remarkable that pulmonary consumption does not so often suspend madness as madness pulmonary consumption."[37] Such observations are made less frequently now, perhaps because tuberculosis is now more effectively treated and does not run its natural course. Certainly, Chekhov left us accounts of his friend I. Levitan's ever-worsening disease—and with it, his paranoid psychotic spells which made caring for him so difficult. There is no clear pattern of "alternation" visible, however.

Anton Pavlovich himself was almost certainly never mad. His periods of depression had at least once led to suicidal thoughts; but that is not psychosis. I mention this particularly because of the interest of his story, "The Black Monk." Chekhov created here a gripping tale of the intellectual Kovrin's tuberculous illness, with its periods of madness alternating with acute physical illness, and with many psychological features of a consumptive's life marvelously described. Chekhov wrote to Suvorin in 1894, "I wrote the 'Black Monk' in no gloomy frame of mind but after cold deliberation. I simply had a desire to describe 'mania grandiosa.' The monk rushing across the field was a dream; on waking in the morning I told it to Misha."[38]

For all its fine evocation of landscape, horticulture, and the portrayal of consumptive and psychotic symptoms, I find the presentation of Kovrin's inner experience of illness disappointing; not quite on target. Is this because Chekhov, uncharacteristically, was approaching his subject so much from the outside in, and not from personal knowledge? Why did he break his own literary rules this way? Was there a personal fear hidden in his fascination with mental illness? And why did he write this story in late 1893, as he was emerging from a year or two of acute episodes of physical illness as well as inner turmoil and unhappiness, and lack of inspiration? I have no answers.

After World War II, research interest burgeoned in the United States and Canada in the psychosomatic aspects of chronic diseases. Our medical forefather, Hippocrates—undistracted by knowledge of bacilli and the exact mechanisms of diseases, in 400 BC—could see very clearly that "Health depends on a state of equilibrium among the various internal factors which govern the operations of the body and the mind."[39] This holistic approach faded in the Enlightenment Age, when body was studied scientifically as separate from mind, and "progress" in the treatment of individual and societal ills was now the goal. In the nineteen fifties, however, many physicians made a new attempt to understand the psychological influences that made a patient vulnerable to a particular disease, or unable to overcome it. Differences in this regard could now be measured to some extent by psychological testing, interviewing in depth, or during psychotherapy. Studies of the lives and test results of tubercular patients in a large hospital, for example, could be contrasted with those of a control group of non-tubercular patients. For tuberculosis, the effective medicine Isonyazid had just become available. It enabled many patients to recuperate and leave the sanatoria. Even then, however, it was not a universal cure. The failure of some patients to benefit was also studied in its physical and psychological aspects.

The book, *Personality, Stress and Tuberculosis*, edited by Dr. Phineas Sparer in 1956, bears witness to this time. Articles there by such remarkable scientists as Hans Selye and E.D. Wittkower of Montreal, Flanders Dunbar of New York, tell of new insights into the impact of stress on tuberculosis; the endocrine functions which are involved in new vulnerability to the bacilli; etc. Except on the bookshelves of psychotherapists treating consumptives, such volumes have largely vanished. Medical progress channeled elsewhere, thunderingly, towards understanding cellular biology, microbial habits, epidemiology. The number of tubercular citizens declined—at least in those parts of the world where sanitation and living conditions could be improved, and medication given and monitored. Cure or improvement by psychotherapy of individuals with chronic disease was more difficult than was hoped. Yes, psychological factors loomed large for many sufferers from consumption, peptic ulcer, lupus erythematosis. But therapeutic intervention in this was often impracticable, and the approach perhaps oversimplified because of still limited knowledge of the intricacies of the "whole person."

I honor these mid-century researchers for their attempt—which may succeed in the future—to bring the holistic insights of Hippocrates and others into the scientific medical mainstream. Anton Chekhov had similar insights. In Russian medical practice, he was even more isolated in this than Drs. Wittkower and Dunbar. He wrote to Suvorin, however, in 1889: "And if you know how great the similarity is between mental and physical illnesses and when you know that both one and the other are treated with the very same remedies, you can't help but refuse to separate soul from body."[40]

To return to our protagonist, the tubercular Anton Chekhov: we might try using some findings of Dr. Wittkower as a background illumination of the place Anton Pavlovich found himself in, in illness.

1. With psychological testing, Dr. Wittkower did find one personality feature to be universal in chronic tubercular patients. "An immoderate need for affection together with conflicts over aggression were found in all the patients studied. The configuration . . . however, depended upon his character defenses developed during childhood. Dependency needs may be freely and unashamedly expressed, may be concealed by a rebellious, hostile front, or may be successfully suppressed."[41]

2. An initial denial of illness is common. When the first symptoms become obvious, many sufferers do not seek medical help. When diagnosed, they refuse to believe it. "*Constructive resignation* is rare in tuberculosis; it is not a disease which any person who realizes its full significance accepts with equanimity."[42] Wittkower describes depression, anxiety, overcheerfulness—and boredom, apathy (that word so frequent in Chekhov's letters)—as frequent reactions. The psychoanalyst Ralph Greenson defined apathy as "a defense against painful perceptions [which] serves the purpose of avoiding overwhelming feelings of annihilation".[43]

3. The chronic patient may carry a powerful sense of aloneness. This may even surpass the chronic alienation of Pavel Chekhov, who had inscribed on his signet ring, "everywhere is a desert to the lonely man." Not only are consumptives often isolated in hospitals and sick rooms: they come to feel that "healthy people" and "sick people" are two exclusive categories. Though they may be visited or even surrounded by healthy friends and family, there is an invisible barrier. Chekhov wrote in his notebook, "As I shall lie in the grave alone, so in fact I live alone." [44]

And there may be a burden of shame and guilt in being chronically ill. I have found no direct expression of this in Chekhov's letters. He was, after all, able to fulfill the family obligation of providing for the others, and bringing them honor, all his adult life. There is a vignette, however, which suggests the presence of guilt. The writer Nemirovich-Danchenko reported that the ailing Chekhov described to him in Nice, the "rows of tuberculous patients lined up on the beach in their chairs, spitting. The sea, healthy, calm and brave rolled towards them. Near the chairs stood the wives and husbands of the sick patients. He would like to write a story, he said, about how these relatives feel, like slaves chained to the galleys."[45]

4. Those patients who allow themselves to face their own condition are pained by the beauty of life. Their own living has no ampleness. The shadow of this feeling passes over again and again, in Anton Pavlovich's correspondence, stories and plays. To his friend Maksim Gorki he said in 1902, "To live in order to die is not amusing, but to live knowing that one must die prematurely is absolutely stupid."[46]

Chekhov's love of amplitude in the world led him to travel, and to buy country estates where he wrote and fished and dug in the gardens. He once described his literary work this way: "...in former times I wrote as a bird sings." And in his notebook he transcribed a quote from Alfonse Daudet.

"'Why are thy songs so short?', a bird was once asked. 'Is it because thou art short of breath?' 'I have very many songs, and I should like to sing them all.'"[47]

In the notebook is a jotting about "a conversation on another planet about the earth a thousand years hence. 'Do you remember that white tree...[silver beech}?'"[48]

"Why do the trees grow and so luxuriously, when the owners are dead?"[49]

As described, the psychosomatic researches of the mid-twentieth-century produced fresh insights into chronic diseases. Hippocrates of the fourth century B.C., and Galen of the second century A.D., had left their corroborating thoughts about the mind/body interconnection. And now Dr. Sigmund Freud had created a widely disseminated theory of the human mind which might illuminate its rich interlacing with the body. For most practicing physicians, however, there was little inclination to consider all this in a live patient's treatment. There were too many patients, too little time — and above all, doctors did not see firm scientific evidence, as they had been trained to demand in making their treatment choices. The linear, repeatable, "proof" of truth set an objective standard that Dr. Chekhov too admired. Thus Koch discovered the bacillus that "caused" tuberculosis, in that it was always present in an active case, if one looked; and if it was present, the illness was ipso facto tuberculosis. Descartes had said in the seventeenth century, leading the Enlightenment views that profoundly influenced medicine, that we will best understand the human body by studying it separately from the mind. It is a "machine so built up and composed of nerves, muscles, veins, blood and skin, that though there were no mind in it at all, it would not cease to have the same [functions]."[50] Until very recently, the chief hope for improvement of patients' care has been placed in developing new techniques for investigating the body; new knowledge of pathological mechanisms even to the intracellular level.

The tools for fine-tuning the treatment of tuberculosis, since Chekhov's day, have multiplied. There came the x-ray, and fluoroscopy, the bronchoscope, the CAT scan, the PET scan; also surgical advancements that made it possible to excise small areas of diseased lung; also, above all, the development of medications. Many, many cases of consumption were arrested and prevented.

Individual chronic sufferers and the newly infected, however, are often disaffected by this approach. They yearn for their minds and souls to be considered in the treatment of their bodies. Some people have turned in recent decades to whatever practitioners of holistic medicine they could find. These doctors try to address the sick person, rather than the diseased body. And they believe that our biomedical model of practice is "after the fact" treatment—just as Dr. Zakharin in 1860's Moscow, and his student Dr. Chekhov, looked to the life conditions of patients and not only to their symptoms. To this date, there has been little everyday translation between the language of the modern scientific and the holistic approaches. Patients must still opt, on trust, for one approach or the other.

Nevertheless, there are intimations now of hope for new integration of these approaches. A "second medical revolution" may be brewing; as basic for change as the first revolution in the seventeenth century. Anton Chekhov would have understood and welcomed this, one hundred years ago. The seminal element for change, this time, is the field of cybernetics.

It has discovered the inadequacy of the simple cause-and-effect, engineering model of thinking about systems, upon which medicine and many other disciplines relied for so long. The "person" is a system. His elements — genetic, biological, cellular, immunological, psychological, historical — are linked as reciprocal influences, and in feedback loops, and to other systems. These include such things as pathogenic bacilli, carcinogens, etc., in the environment: each with its own system, feeding back and wielding influence. A disturbance in the equilibrium between a person's and his surroundings' systems causes 'disease' in him. A study of all these elements and interconnections can locate the point of breakdown. The targeted treatment made possible can be vastly more successful.

As with the stirrings of the Russian revolution-to-come in the late nineteenth and early twentieth centuries — what the future change will look like cannot be predicted. This new approach is also a system. What will the influences of politics and economics alone be, to foster it or wither it, in the practice of medicine? There is promise, surely, if it is not extinguished, for better medical care. The physician could gather a wide variety of pertinent information about the patient that would be both "scientific" and believable for them both. Doctor and patient could more trustingly and equally, then, settle on the right choices to restore health. In tuberculosis, it is helpful to see that the presence of the Koch bacillus is essential, but not its single "cause." Nor is the psychological state of the patient. The word "cause" can be redefined.

None of this would have been new to Dr. Chekhov except the burgeoning theory and technology of this later time. He listened well to patients and was an excellent diagnostician. To these habits, too, we owe the wonderful accuracy — and open-mindedness — of his depiction of men and women in his stories and plays.

One of his medical advisories to his friend Suvorin is old - fashioned in its medications, but well targeted and holistic. "Swaying, reeling accompanied by dimness of vision or even loss of consciousness for a few seconds . . . is a phenomenon that is almost usual in men of your age . . . One must come to terms with it . . . Don't walk too quickly when your brain is working or when wearing a heavy overcoat. It is a common illness in elderly peasants and I treat it by saying that they should not be frightened and should not change their mode of life. In addition I give them valerian, ten drops four times a day especially if the pulse is weak. Every case is treated on its merits."[51]

There might, or might not, come a day when the art and the science of medicine are more collaborative. Certainly, some scientists will always work best within the walls of the laboratory, while others come forth, with an intuitive talent, to work with patients. Anton Chekhov as person was a complex system. He liked to work as a doctor in both the above ways. Yet he needed his mistress, literature, and did not want her in the same household with his medical "wife."

He did thrive on separations; alternations. He kept an equilibrium that was delicate but sturdy, most of the time. But many inner and outer systems during his life malfunctioned. There was unlucky, debilitating feedback that fed his consumptive illness.

VI.
Anton Chekhov Was Here

On an April morning in Moscow, Dr. Z, junior physician, is bringing a discharge form to a patient for signature. The departing patient is Anton Pavlovich Chekhov, who entered the Ostroumov Clinic near the Novodevichie Cemetery in March. Dr. Z is wearing a perfectly fresh white coat. The bell of his stethoscope pokes up emblematically from a side pocket. He is a rather short man, well-built and limber. Only somewhat sunshine deprived and tired looking. On his face one sees various mingling emotions: his features are more mobile and self-revealing than those of most young postdoctoral physicians. His slender nose, with flaring nostrils, is especially expressive. Since matriculating at Moscow University Medical School, he has been able to conceal his mouth in a full black bushy beard, however. Right now, he is adjusting his face to near impassivity. He knocks at the door of a far room on the corridor of Ward 16. A soft male voice calls, "Come in."

Here is a big, white, very bright room with a white bed, a big white table, a little cupboard and some chairs.[1] Dr. Z always likes to attend patients in this airy and civilized space. Being on the sunny garden side, it is kept by Dr. Ostroumov for the most eminent patients at his clinic, and is frequently empty. Dr. Chekhov is sitting in the large bedside chair. He is fully dressed. Dr. Z has expected that, knowing that Ivan Pavlovich Chekhov has promised to come and carry his brother home at eleven. But Dr. Z has previously seen Chekhov only in hospital robe and nightshirt. The carefully knotted black tie, the frockcoat, the cufflinks in a starched white shirt, are elegant but off-putting. So are the black hat and thick wool overcoat laid out neatly on the bed. Dr. Chekhov's pince-nez are on his nose. The ribbon attached to them is sternly black. This patient looks more old and thin and ill in full dress than in hospital robe: that is disconcerting to his young doctor.

A pile of papers and books that enlivened and personalized the white table for two weeks is gone. A small valise with gold clasps stands closed, waiting beside the chair. It seems to have swallowed all the things from Anton Pavlovich's world which he'd spread out here awhile. *Futliar* — envelope, case, opaque container — is the word that passes through Dr. Z's mind. He is disappointed. He had hoped that their conversation of last evening might continue a little. But Dr. Chekhov only nods, doesn't smile, and returns his gaze to a bare beech tree branch that bobs outside the window. Dr. Z glances at it too. The branch informs them that the wind is gusting; that sunlight can define all things beautifully; that Spring is coming to Moscow but is not yet here. Dr. Z notches up his impassivity a bit more. "Here is the discharge paper, sir. Please sign, for the hospital record." He detaches a sheet of paper clipped to a bulky folder he is carrying. Anton Pavlovich smiles faintly, and reaches out a slender hand for the document. Now he's indeed recognized the young man. "A concise ending to the story, is it?" he teases him, in that frail voice. "This two-week-long story of me you hold under your arm?"

Dr. Z blushes. He has read this "story" so many times that it's almost memorized. Does Anton Chekhov perceive that? Actually, it was Z who wrote a good deal of it. He entered the daily vital signs. He recorded the physical examinations done by the senior staff. He himself elicited from Dr. Chekhov the family history of his disease, and the environmental and social aspects that might have bearing. Anton Pavlovich Chekhov is the favorite patient so far of his medical career. He has also been his favorite author since gymnasia days. He himself wrote one story at seventeen with a Chekhovian flavor. In his leisure reading at University he had to give up Tolstoy and Turgenev and most of the others, for lack of time. Chekhov he kept; reading each new piece as it came out in *Russian Thought* or the *Russian Gazette*.

Anton Pavlovich has turned to the table to dip a pen into the inkwell and write. There is, alas, nothing more for Dr.Z to say or do. The difference in their coats, neckties, ages, seem to dash his hopes that there will be a real parting handshake.

While Dr. Chekhov finishes signing, there is a firm knock on the room door, and it is opened without ceremony. In comes a tall, vigorous man. He looks around at the belongings in the room, and at their owner — offers a quick nod to Dr. Z — then turns wholly to Anton. Now Dr. Z can scan him openly. Striking how much he resembles Dr. Chekhov: the cut of the well trimmed beard; a certain look in the eyes. But younger, and less highly focused. Healthy.

Anton Pavlovich is holding the signed discharge paper in his hand.

"Vanya," he says, in a slightly stronger voice than Dr.Z has heard. "Everything is ready."

"Good", says Vanya. "Were you able to gather the money? Masha says we need it at once — there's none at home."

Anton nods, and looks amused as well as tired.

"And put on your overcoat, it's cold out there. Probably *very* cold at home today."

Dr. Chekhov hands the signed sheet to Dr. Z, who is hovering near. "Goodbye" is imminent. But Vanya — in charge here at the moment — is just telling Anton that they'll have to stop by in the carriage to buy pork breast and candles, on the way to the train. Anton is listening in a semi-cheerful way. Vanya keeps talking. Anton is reaching for his hat; enlivened, beginning to look feisty and a little contemptuous. Z — an only child — is placed right for intimate witness to the older brother's and the younger's sparring and dealing. Like a very young brother, he draws back and gawks. He forgets the attention he'd wanted himself. Eventually, Dr. Chekhov shakes Dr. Z's hand limply, and briefly meets his eyes, but is not really looking. Anton Pavlovich seems to have left this place already — gone home to his family. Dr. Z leaves the room quietly.

He walks the corridor to the ward office. He'll at least take time to study Dr. Chekhov's signature there, before entering the sheet into the chart. Then when he is off duty, he can mull again all details of last evening. They can be stored in his mind; always available for recall.

In the early evening of yesterday he had accompanied Dr. A and Dr. B to Anton Pavlovich's room. There must be a final physical examination of Dr. Chekhov, and any further serious discussion needed about the prognosis and the recommended medical care. Dr.Z knew that his senior colleagues were feeling their responsibility. Dr. Ostroumov happened to be away at Sukhum on the Black Sea, when this famous man was brought unexpectedly to his Moscow clinic. Ostroumov's juniors, A and B, were excellent and experienced physicians. They knew thoroughly by now Ostroumov's particular techniques of auscultation and percussion, the details of up-to-date treatment of phthisis, and all the perspectives on tuberculosis which Ostroumov championed. A touch of stage fright, only, showed itself in their especially brusque and determined approach to Anton Pavlovich's door. Z, as the most junior physician, would have no say in this visit; only carried the chart.

Dr. Chekhov was sitting in the bedside chair, wearing a white hospital dressing gown. He seemed to have finished supper — though on the tray on the table was considerable uneaten food. He nursed a half-empty wineglass in his hands.

"Gentlemen . . ." He waved them in.

“Dr. Chekhov.” Dr. A led the delegation to the bedside. “If supper is over, may we examine you once more — and tie up all loose ends.”

Anton Pavlovich waved a languid acceptance. Dr. Z came forward to remove the tray to a spot near the door; as seriously as he assists in the operating room. He received the wine glass from Anton’s hand. Dr. A had meanwhile scanned the food left on the plate. “You have fine food here. Is that woodcock? But still you eat poorly. Your weight is very little better.” All present knew that Dr. A disapproved of Chekhov’s eating habits, and also of his friends’ bringing him delicacies not on the hospital menu. He had expressed all this several times. But Dr. Chekhov seemed oblivious. “I prefer roast chicken. But it gives me erotic dreams — it’s better to sleep.” He smiled faintly.

“Here now.” Drs. A and B combined to free Chekhov’s upper body from the dressing gown. Now he sat on the side of the bed in the skimpy hospital gown. He looked skimpy himself; pale; much older than his thirty-seven years. Dr. A first studied the patient’s neck and torso, front and back, with a focused clinical eye. Dr.Z, watching, thought about Dr. A’s age: thirty-three. And Dr. B, second in authority to A, was already forty. B would have graduated three years before Chekhov. Still, at this vulnerable moment, Anton Pavlovich could easily be taken for their frail uncle or father.

Now Dr. A began to percuss the left side of Dr. C’s chest: top to bottom, front and back, then the right side. The sturdy third finger of his left hand was the drum, sliding along smoothly and efficiently. The pounding finger of his right hand was the drumstick.

Z thought, watching him, that all the delicacy and art of this gruff man is concentrated in the fingers. “Take in a breath — hold it please.” “Now exhale.” (The wheezing exhalations could be heard across the room.) Then without turning his head, Dr. A began reciting his findings to Dr. Z as he went along. Dr. Z was quite ready, with a pencil and a small notebook pulled from his breast pocket.

"A moderate hollow below the left clavicle", said Dr. A. "Depressed breath sounds above, and extending three centimeters below. Occasional rales front and back, left upper. Frequent expiratory rhonchi over both lungs front and back; most marked on left."

Dr. Z jotted it all down. Nothing was a surprise; the same findings were noted at Anton Pavlovich's admission physical two weeks ago. Only the hemorrhages since had been fewer and shorter.

Dr. B took his turn, repeating the procedures of Dr. A. At the end he told Dr. Z — "agreed in all details." Z wrote. Before this jotting, he had had time to let his thoughts stray. His eyes had wandered to the pile of letters, papers — perhaps stories? — and books, perching on top of Anton Chekhov's cupboard . . . magical. Then he'd reflected that if this were an ordinary patient, not one so special to Dr. Ostroumov, he would be having his turn too at the percussion and auscultation. Junior staff is usually encouraged to learn... however, would he have wished to lay his fingers on Anton Chekhov's chest in this way? To bend down his head so close to Anton Pavlovich Chekhov, moving the bell of his stethoscope here and there, over the skin of the author whose work he reveres? Drs. A and B showed no such diffidence. Z would not have expected it of them. They plainly do not consider writers to have the importance of doctors of medicine. Some evenings ago, when Lev Tolstoy visited Chekhov and stayed so overlong, and Chekhov had the serious hemorrhage that night, they cursed this "overblown Tolstoy" at breakfast. Understandable. But even Mikhail, their illiterate old peasant gatekeeper at the Clinic door, told Dr. Z with Russian pride about the imperial awesome arrival of the famous Tolstoy. Enormous white beard!! Even Matron, who'd entered Anton Pavlovich's room at eight o'clock that evening and found Tolstoy still there, talking and talking — "outrageous!" — told them at lunch, with awe and contempt, that the men seemed ready to argue all night about "whether you go somewhere after you die or if you don't, or some such." The young man suddenly realized that he was despising these doctors whom he ordinarily respects. He felt utterly sick of all this medical intrusion on another human being's physical dignity. This power to alter the course of a life!

His thoughts were interrupted by the half opening of the room's door — with no preceding knock. The head and shoulders of a very pretty young woman appeared: ash blonde hair showing around the edges of her white cap. The starched blue-striped shawl collar of a junior nurse identified her, and looked most becoming. Her eyes sparkled in the direction of Anton Pavlovich. Her mouth was already open in anticipation, to speak, to laugh; as though there'd been only a brief interruption in some lively conversation. But immediately, she saw the situation. She picked up Dr. Chekhov's tray from the floor with intense professionalism, and vanished with it through the doorway. Only Z, and C, had seen her. Chekhov's eyes were twinkling a little. He'd sat up straighter.

Now the senior doctors helped Chekhov into his robe again. Dr. A sat down in the bedside chair, and leafed through the patient's chart. Then he spoke very bluntly to Anton Pavlovich.

"There's been no essential change from the beginning. The three positive sputums leave no doubt of the diagnosis. Dr. Ostroumov sent word — you're to think of yourself as a sick man, from here on in. 'Crippled', he put it. That's the way it is. Please be careful, be cautious — don't overdo. Peace. Nutrition. You say you don't like koumiss; we highly recommend it nevertheless. And as we've discussed, a dry climate by this winter. Mediterranean, Crimea. Leave Moscow and Melikhovo by October at the latest. And subcutaneous arsenic for the next month. Agreed?"

Chekhov was studying Dr. A's face as he talked. He nodded noncommittally. Dr. A did not press for verbal agreement. He had discharged his duty; now summoned up a fairly cordial handshake for his patient on leaving. Followed by Dr. B, he went from the room.

Dr. Z would stay a few moments longer, to transcribe his penciled notes into the record. He could add a short paragraph of summary narrative using the pen and inkstand on Dr.Chekhov's table; the ones Anton Chekhov has used.

Both men were silent. Anton Pavlovich spoke first, quietly. "Are you enjoying the clinic?"

Dr. Z. closed the chart, "Oh, very much. I'm one of the lucky ones — learning from Dr. Ostroumov. The best!" He recaptured the savor of his new career at once, with deep pleasure. "The best . . .", Dr. Chekhov echoed in his softer, paler voice; trailed off, but then added, "Yes. A fine man. A brave one too."

Both nodded. "I wrote my clinical case history for him, in the last year of University. It was Zakharin I loved, though — as you love Ostroumov. You knew Zakharin too?"

"No. Oh, of course we all recognized him, passing in the corridor and such. You know, the first year students still can't attend the lectures of the great men."(Z shook his head.) "Then in 1894, just when I reached the clinical years, there were those terrible accusations against him. He had to resign." The two men looked somberly at each other.

"Dreadful," said Anton Pavlovich. Then he changed the subject.

"Where are you from? Wait, let me guess. Voronezh, perhaps?"

Dr. Z's eyes widened. "Close! How did you know? Zadonsk, only kilometers away."

Chekhov laughed, mouth open, eyes lighting. (He has eyes like a dachshund, Dr. Z decided. His own family has three dachshunds; all, even in their old age, with bright, intelligent, contemplative eyes.) "I am famous for my telepathic knowledge . . . no, really, it is the shape of your nose. I was once in Voronezh at the St. Alexey Monastery, to hear the beautiful singing. I noticed so many slender, expressive noses on the faces in the congregation." He laughed merrily. Then coughed awhile, and spat; and quieted.

"What will you do next? Will you stay at this clinic?"

"I'm not sure. I'll probably take a zemstvo position — the Moscow zemstvo, I know its the most progressive. That's the only good choice for a doctor now, conditions are so bad. Social medicine is the only way to press for change." Dr. Z spoke with some passion. He broke off, however, feeling he'd forgotten it was A.P. Chekhov to whom he was speaking. Dr. Chekhov had made quite different professional choices.

He backtracked a little in his confusion. "Private practice would make a good wide field of action, too," he said, "but I can't afford it. They say there's poor pay or *no* pay in the provinces. And I haven't the connections for Moscow or St. Petersburg. Really, I don't have the flair for the wealthy patients, either. I'd end up a poor drunk! They'd bury me early."

The young man was urgently wishing for Dr. Chekhov's advice. It would feel childish to ask for it. He might receive unasked advice, however: Dr C was really engaged in this conversation. Anton Pavlovich's face was alight again — just as the young nurse had lighted it.

But Anton said unexpectedly: "I see you are also a writer." A smiling, teasing expression.

Dr. Z blushed deep red, from neck to hairline.

"Forgive me, just a hunch. Sometimes I see things in people's faces."

"Well . . .yes . . . no. I used to like to write. Short stories, and poems, in gymnasia days. But I've really fallen in love with medicine. Everything now goes there. It takes all of me."

Chekhov nodded. “I understand. Best not to chase two hares, probably. That’s what they tell *me*. Be an Ostroumov — or a Zakharin. All power to you! For me, two hares were necessary. I can’t explain why — but it’s agreed with me.”

They looked cordially at each other, then a touch ruefully, as they both contemplated Chekhov’s words. Then very quickly, Anton Pavlovich’s optimism faded away. He let his slippers drop off his feet to the floor. He laid himself back onto his pillow. “I’m quite tired,” he said.

“Goodnight, sir.” Dr. Z lowered the wick of the table lamp: just a dim light so the night nurse could see. He went quietly, out into the corridor. As he walked now, he planned, “I might drop in for a minute after his breakfast tomorrow, and before the brother comes for him. There’ll be the discharge sheet to sign. I’ll take it in myself.”

ENDNOTES

Preface (pp. 7-10)

1. Charles du Bos, "The Chekhovian Sense of Life," in Robert L. Jackson's *Chekhov, a Collection of Critical Essays,* pp. 190-191.
2. Maksim Gorky, "Reminiscences of Tchekhov," in Koteliansky and Woolf's *Anton Tchekhov's Notebooks with Reminiscences of Tchekhov by Maxim Gorky,* p.97.
3. A.P. Chekhov, letter to Alexei S. Suvorin, Nov. 20, 1888.

Chapter I (pp. 11-20)

1. As described by Kolya Chekhov in *Childhood Reminiscences,* 1889. Quoted by Donald Rayfield in *Anton Chekhov, a Life,* p. 10.
2. Pavel Chekhov, letter to A.P. Chekhov, 1876.
3. As described by Olga Knipper-Tchekhova in "Tchekhov's Last Hours," in Koteliansky and Tomlinson's *The Life and Letters of Anton Tchekhov* , p. 304.

Chapter II (pp. 21-30)

1. Simon Karlinsky in *Letters of Anton Chekhov,* p. 32.
2. A.P. Chekhov, letter to A.S. Suvorin, April 8, 1892.
3. Maria Chekhova in a memoir quoted by D. Rayfield in *Anton Chekhov, a Life,* p. 205.
4. D. Rayfield in *Anton Chekhov, a Life,* p. 453.

Chapter III (pp. 31-49)

1. A.P. Chekhov, letter to Dr. Grigori Rossolimo, Oct. 11, 1899.
2. N. Frieden in *Russian Physicians in an Era of Reform and Revolution, 1856-1905*, p. 13.
3. A.P. Chekhov in Koteliansky and Woolf's *Anton Tchekhov's Note-books*, p. 81.
4. A.P .Chekhov, letter to A.S. Suvorin, Dec. 24, 1890.
5. V. Veresaeff, in *The Confessions of a Physician*, p. 1.
6. Ibid., p. 4.
7. Ibid., p. 44.
8. Ibid., p. 43.
9. Ibid., p. 169.
10. Ibid., p. 147.
11. Ibid., p. 194.
12. Ibid., p. 131.
13. A.P. Chekhov, quoted by V.V. Khizniakov in *Anton Pavlovich Chekhov kak vrach*, Moscow 1947, p. 127.
14. A.P. Chekhov in *Uncle Vanya*, Penguin Classics Edition of Chehov plays, 1959, pp. 187-8.
15. A.P. Chekhov, letter to Aleksandr Chekhov, May 13, 1883.
16. A.P. Chekhov, letter to A.S. Suvorin, Oct. 27, 1888.
17. A.P. Chekhov, letter to A.S. Suvorin, May 30, 1888.
18. A.P. Chekhov, letter to A.S. Suvorin, May 30, 1888.
19. A.P. Chekhov, letter to A.S. Suvorin, March 9, 1890.
20. Mikhail P. Chekhov, in his biographical notes on A.P. Chekhov published by E.B. Meve in Ch. 4 of *Meditsina v tvorchestve i zhizni A.P.Chekhova*, Moscow. Quoted by J. Coope in *Doctor Chekhov*, p. 100.
21. V.F. Snegirev, in 1898 eulogy of Prof. Zakharin. Quoted by J Coope, in *Doctor Chekhov*, pp.125-6.
22. A.P. Chekhov, letter to A.S. Suvorin, August, 1892.
23. A.P.Chekhov, letter to A.S. Suvorin, August 16, 1892.
24. A.P.Chekhov, letter to A.S. Suvorin, August 18, 1891.

25. Maria Chekhova, quoted in E.B. Meve, op. cit., p.15; cited in J. Coope, *Doctor Chekhov,* p. 111.

Chapter IV (pp. 50-70)

1. D. Rayfield in *Anton Chekhov, a Life* , p.4.
2. A.P. Chekhov as quoted in N.M. Ezhov's memoir of 1909.
3. Aleksandr Chekhov, letter to Maria Chekhova in 1890's.
4. Efim Efimiev, quoted by D .Rayfield in *Anton Chekhov, a Life,* p. 17.
5. A.P. Chekhov, letter to Aleksandr Chekhov, January 2, 1889.
6. A.P. Chekhov, letter to Mikhail M. Chekhov, May 10, 1877.
7. A.P. Chekhov, letter to A.S. Suvorin, June 16, 1892.
8. A.P. Chekhov, letter to A.S. Suvorin, Oct. 17, 1889.
9. Lika Mizinova, letter to A.P. Chekhov, 1892.
10. D.V. Grigorovich, letter to A.S. Suvorin, 1889.
11. A. Gruzinsky, letter to N.M. Ezhov, Dec. 1888 or January 1889.
12. A.P. Chekhov to A.S. Suvorin, Jan.7, 1889.
13. A.P. Chekhov, letter to A. Plescheev, Oct. 4, 1888.
14. C. du Bos, "The Chekhovian Sense of Life", in R.L. Jackson, *Chekhov, a Collection of Critical Essays,* p.187
15. A.P. Chekhov, letter to Nikolai P. Chekhov, March, 1886.
16. A.P. Chekhov, letter to A.S. Suvorin, May 28, 1891.
17. A.P. Chekhov, letter to A.S. Suvorin, Sept. 11, 1888.
18. A.P. Chekhov, letter to N.A. Leykin, May 27, 1886.
19. A.P. Chekhov, letter to A.S. Suvorin, September 11, 1888.
20. C. du Bos, "The Chekhovian Sense of Life", in R.L.Jackson, *Chekhov, a Collection of Critical Essays,* p. 192.

21. A.P. Chekhov ,letter to A.S. Suvorin, Dec. 27, 1889.
22. A.P. Chekhov, letter to Nikolai Chekhov, March, 1886.
23. A.P. Chekhov, letter to A.S. Suvorin, September 11, 1888.
24. A.P. Chekhov, letter to A.S. Suvorin, August 16, 1892.
25. A.P. Chekhov, letter to A.S. Suvorin, June 27, 1890.
26. A.P. Chekhov, letter to A.S. Suvorin, August 16, 1892.
27. A.P. Chekhov, letter to A.S. Suvorin, December 1, 1895.
28. A.P. Chekhov, letter to Ivan P. Chekhov, March 5, 1892.
29. A.P. Chekhov, letter to A.S. Suvorin, August 16, 1892.
30. Liodor Palmin, letter to A.P.Chekhov quoted by D. Rayfield in *Anton Chekhov, a Life*, p.103.
31. A.P. Chekhov, letter to Alexandr Chekhov, April, 1883.
32. A.P. Chekhov, letter to A.S. Suvorin, May 30, 1888.
33. A.P. Chekhov, letter to Maria Kiselyova, January 14, 1887.
34. Dr. Pavel Archangelsky quoted in E.B. Meve, op. cit., p. 70; cited by J. Coope in *Doctor Chekhov* , p.27.
35. E.B. Meve, op. cit., p. 15; cited by J. Coope in *Doctor Chekhov* ,p. 111.
36. N. Teleshev, *Reminiscences,* 1943 , pp.101-2; cited in J.Coope's *Doctor Chekhov,* pp. 11-12.
37. A.P. Chekhov, letter to G. Rossolimo, October 11, 1899.

Chapter V (pp.71-89)

1. A.P. Chekhov, letter to A. Pleshcheev, October 4, 1888.
2. A.P. Chekhov, letter to A.S. Suvorin, October 14, 1888.
3. A.P. Chekhov, letter to A. Pleshcheev, October 4, 1888.
4. A.P. Chekhov, letter to A.S. Suvorin,1890.
5. A.P. Chekhov, letter to A.S. Suvorin, Dec. 9, 1890.

6. A.P. Chekhov, letter to A.S. Suvorin, Sept. 8, 1891.

7. A.P. Chekhov, letter to A.S. Suvorin, Nov. 18, 1891.

8. A.P. Chekhov, letter to A.S. Suvorin, Nov. 22, 1891.

9. A.P. Chekhov, letter to Alexandr Smagin, Dec. 1891.

10. A.P. Chekhov, letter to A.S. Suvorin, August, 1893.

11. A. P.Chekhov, letter to Aleksandr Chekhov, April 15, 1894.

12. Jean Schleglov, *A.P.Chekhov, his literary customs and his work*, 1928, p. 285.

13. Prof. M.M. Kovalevsky, December 18, 1897, quoted in *Polnoe sobranie sochinenii i pisem* (PSSP), 7, 517. Quoted in D. Rayfield, *Anton Chekhov, a Life*, p. 445.

14. A.S. Suvorin; see *Novoe vremia* , no. 1017, July 4, 1904. Quoted in D.Rayfield, *Anton Chekhov, a Life*, p. 244.

15. A.P. Chekhov to Lidia Avilova, quoted in D. Rayfield, *Anton Chekhov, a Life*, p.460.

16. A.P. Chekhov, letter to G. Rossolimo, Oct. 11, 1899.

17. A.P.Chekhov, letter to Fiodor Dmitrievich Batiushkov, January, 1900.

18. A.P. Chekhov letter to Lidia Avilova, 1900.

19. A.P.Chekhov, letter to Konstantin Dmitrievich Balmont, January, 1902.

20. A.P.Chekhov, letter to Olga Knipper-Chekhova, 1903.

21. Ivan Alekseevich Bunin, in memoir of A.P. Chekhov, describing visit to Chekhov in Yalta, 1903.

22. A.P. Chekhov, letter to Lidia Avilova, 1904.

23. A.P. Chekhov, letter to Maria Chekhova, June 6, 1904.

24. A.P. Chekhov, letter to Maria Chekhova, June, 1904.

25. A.P. Chekhov, letter to Maria Chekhova, June 28, 1904.

26. A.P. Chekhov, letter to Franz Schechtel, 1896.

27. Rene and Jean Dubos, *The White Plague: Tuberculosis, Man and Society*, pp. 44-65.

28. Susan Sontag, *AIDS and its Metaphors*, p.13.

29. Susan Sontag, *Illness as Metaphor*, p.26-35.

30. Franz Kafka as quoted in S. Sontag's *Illness as Metaphor*, p.43.

31. E.D. Wittkower, M.D., "Psychological Aspects of Pulmonary Tuberculosis", in *Personality, Stress and Tuberculosis,* P.J. Sparer, M.D., Ed., p. 155.

32. E.D. Wittkower, M.D., op.cit., p.155.

33. E.D. Wittkower, M.D., op.cit., p. 156.

34. E.D. Wittkower, M.D.,op.cit., p. 155.

35. Ibid., p. 156.

36. Ibid., p. 157.

37. Dr. Benjamin Rush, quoted by E.D. Wittkower, M.D., "Psychological Aspects of Pulmonary Tuberculosis", in *Personality, Stress and Tuberculosis,* P.J.Sparer, M.D., Ed., p.153.

38. A.P. Chekhov, letter to A.S. Suvorin, January 25, 1894.

39. Hippocrates, quoted by Rene Dubos in *Mirage of Health*, 1959, p. 114.

40. A.P. Chekhov, letter to A.S. Suvorin, May 7, 1889.

41. E.D. Wittkower, M.D., op. cit., p.157.

42. E.D. Wittkower,M.D., op.cit.,p. 163.

43. R.R. Greenson M.D., "The Psychology of Apathy," in *Psychoanalytic Quarterly*, 18, 290-302.

44. A.P. Chekhov in Koteliansky and Woolf's *Anton Tchekhov's Notebooks*, p.49.

45. A.P . Chekhov in conversation with V.I. Nemirovich-Danchenko. Quote from E.B. Meve, op. cit., Ch. 4; as cited by J. Coope in *Doctor Chekhov,* pp.142-3.

46. A.P. Chekhov in conversation with M. Gorki, 1902. Quote from V.V. Knizniakov, *Anton Pavlovich Chekhov kak vrach* ,1947, p.51, cited by J. Coope in *Doctor Chekhov*, p. 151.

47. A.P. Chekhov in Koteliansky and Woolf's *Anton Chekhov's Notebooks*,p.26.

48. Ibid., p. 38.

49. Ibid., p.47.

50. Rene Descartes in *Traite de L'homme;* quoted in L. Foss and K. Rothenberg, *The Second Medical Revolution*, p.24.

51. A.P. Chekhov, letter to A. S. Suvorin, October 17, 1892.

Chapter VI (pp. 90-99)

1. Chekhov's room in the Ostroumov Clinic was described approximately this way by Olga Shavrova, in a wire she sent to her sister Elena on March 29, 1897, after visiting Anton. Quoted by D. Rayfield in *Anton Chekhov, a Life*, p. 424.

BIBLIOGRAPY

Anderson, Janet M. "Ellen Emerson and the Tubercular Muse"; in *Literature and Medicine*,Vol. 18, #1, Spring, 1999, pp. 39-59.

Berlin, Isaiah. *Russian Thinkers*. New York: Hogarth Press, 1978.

Bunin, I.A. *O Chekhove*. New York: 1955.

Chekhov as Remembered by his Contemporaries. Moscow: 1960.

Chekhov, A.P. *Izbrannye proizvedeniya v trekh tomakh*. Moscow: Izdatelstvo Khudogestvennaya literatura, 1964.

Chekhov, A.P. *Ostrov Sakhalin*. English translation in *Journey to Sakhalin*, 1993.

Chekhov Plays. Penguin Classics English edition, introduction by Elizaveta Fen; London: Whitefriars Press, 1959.

Chekhova, Maria. *Pisma k bratu A.P.Chekhovu*. Moscow: 1954.

Chekhova, Maria. *Iz daliokogo proshlogo*. Moscow: 1960.

Coope, Dr. John. *Doctor Chekhov, a Study in Literature and Medicine*. Isle of Wight: Cross Publishing, 1997.

de Maegd-Soëp, Carolina. *Chekhov and Women in the Life and Work of Chekhov*. Ohio: 1987.

Dubos, Rene and Jean. *The White Plague: Tuberculosis, Man and Society*. New York: Little Brown, 1952.

Dubos, Rene. *The Mirage of Health*. New York: Little Brown, 1959.

Foss, Lawrence and Rothenberg, Kenneth. *The Second Medical Revolution*. New Science Library, Shambhal Publications; Random House distrib. in U.S., 1987.

Frieden, Nancy. *Russian Physicians in an Era of Reform and Revolution, 1856-1905*. New Jersey: Princeton University Press, 1981.

Garnet, Constance. *Letters of Anton Chekhov to Family and Friends*. 1920 (C.G.'s translation and biog. sketch).

Jackson, Robert L., Editor. *Chekhov, a Collection of Critical Essays*. New Jersey: Prentice Hall, 1967.

Karlinsky, Simon, with Henry Heim. *Letters of Anton Chekhov*. New York: Harper and Row, 1973.

Koteliansky, S.S. - Edit., and Trans. with Tomlinson. *The Life and Letters of Anton Tchekhov*. London: Cassell and Co., 1925.

Koteliansky, S.S. *Anton Chekhov, Literary and Theatrical Reminiscences*, London: Routledge and Kegan Paul, 1927.

Koteliansky, S.S. and Leonard Woolf. Trans., *The Notebooks of Anton Tchekhov together with Reminiscences of Tchekhov by Maxim Gorky*. Hogarth Press, 1921.

Literaturnoe nasledstvo 68: Chekhov. Moscow: 1960.

Pritchett, V.S. *Chekhov, a Spirit Set Free*. New York: Random House, 1988.

Psychoanalytic Quarterly, vol. 18, New York.

Rayfield, Donald. *Anton Chekhov, a Life*. London: Harper Collins, 1997.

Sontag, Susan. *Illness as Metaphor*. New York: Farrar, Strauss and Giroux, 1979.

Sontag, Susan. *AIDS and its Metaphors*. New York: Farrar, Strauss and Giroux, 1988.

Sparer, Dr. Phineas J., Edit. *Personality, Stress and Tuberculosis*. New York: International Universities Press, 1956.

Veresaeff, V. (pseudonym of Smidovich, V.). *The Confessions of a Physician*; English translation by Simeon Linden. New York: Frederick A. Stokes, 1904.

INDEX

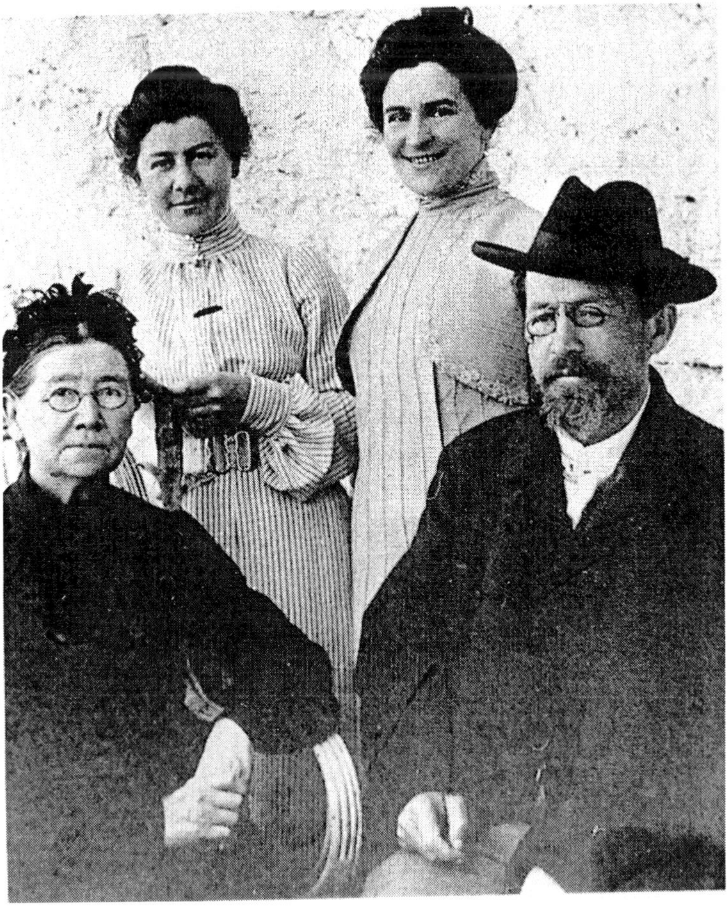

Chekhov with his family: mother, Evgeniia Iakovlevna Chekhova, sister, Mariia Pavlovna Chekhova, wife, Olga Leonardovna Knipper-Chekova (Yalta, Febr. 1902)

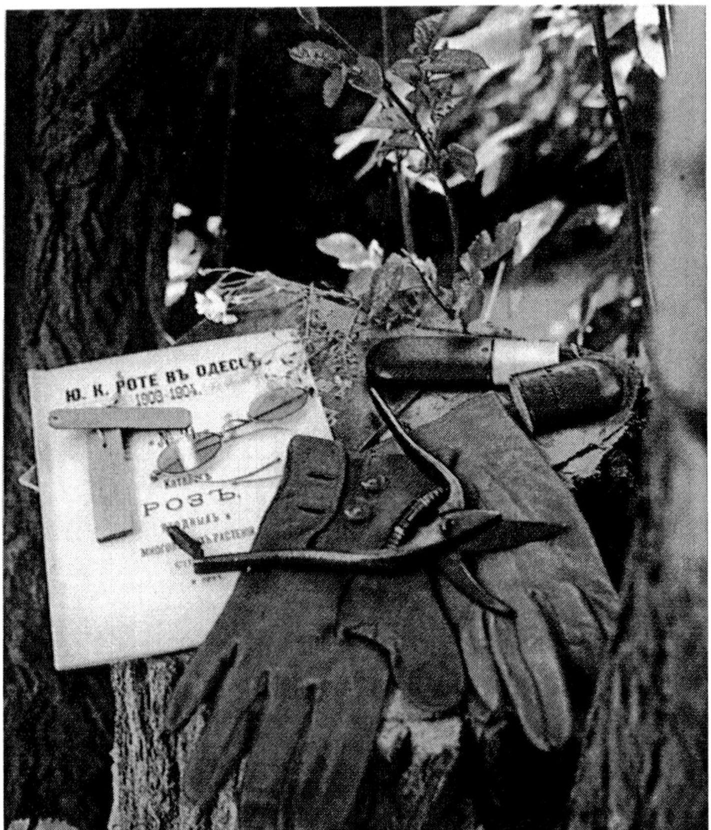

Chekhov’s garden tools

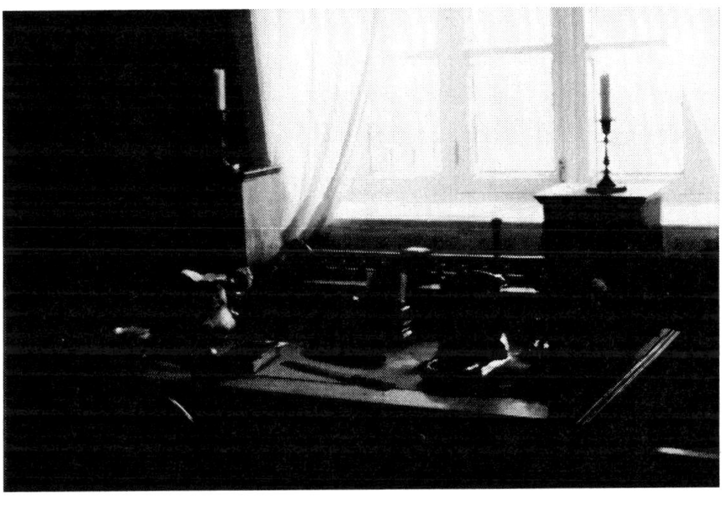

Chekhov's writing desk in Yalta

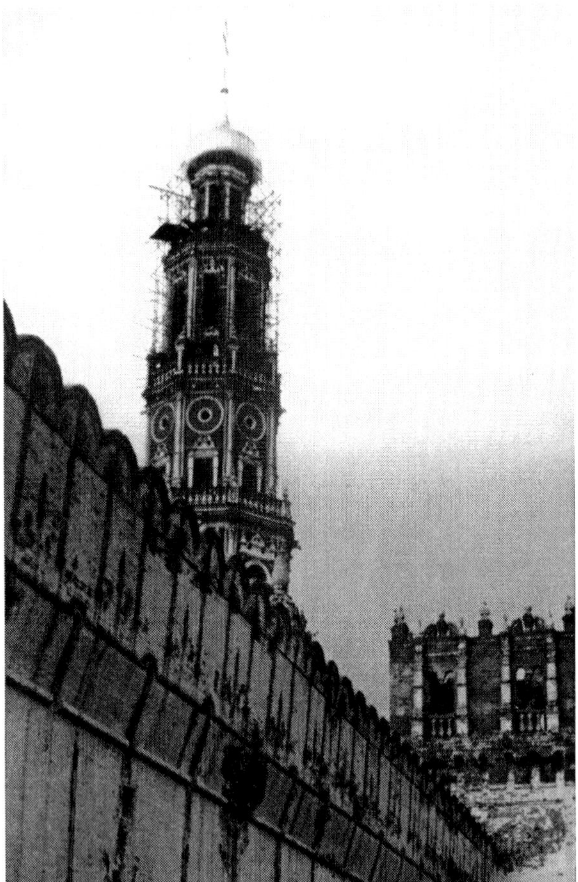

Novodevichii Monastery in Moscow where Chekhov was buried

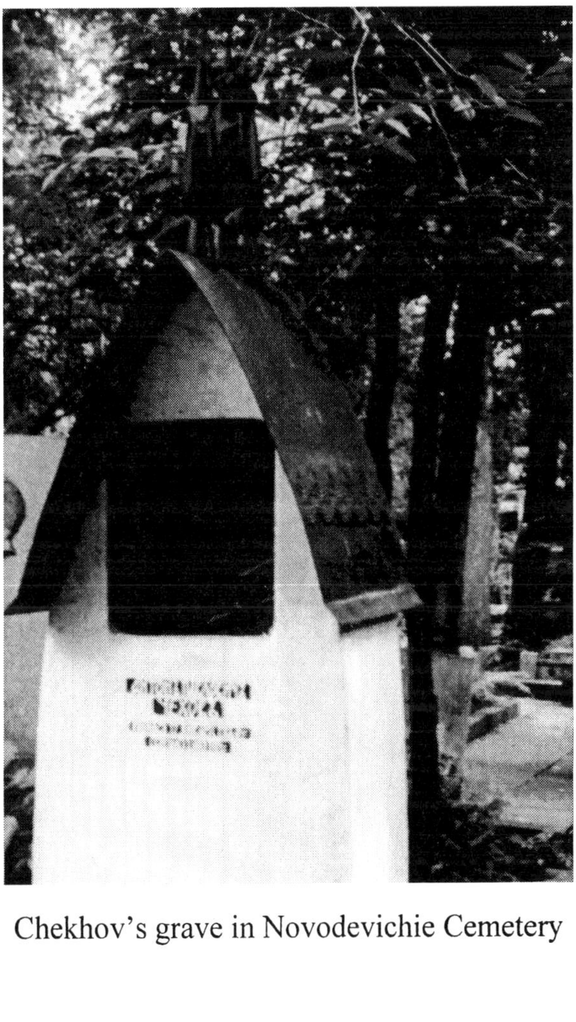

Chekhov's grave in Novodevichie Cemetery